THE FOOD SOLUTION

Skip the Chemically Ridden Altered Products (C.R.A.P.).
Start Your 21-Day Diet Detox Today and Thrive.

Cari Schaefer, M.A., TCM, L.Ac.

ACKNOWLEDGMENTS

I am forever grateful to all the people who have supported me on my journey. But I want to mention a few people who have played a pivotal role in my completing this book. My teachers, mentors, and friends: Dr. Jeannette & George Birnbach, Dr. Deb & Scott Walker, Dr. Freddie Ulan & Dr. Lester Bryman, Tom Van Dyke, Scott Coady, my Mom and Grandfather, my beloved Jonathon, Shannon, Sascha, my dear friends who have listened to me talk about it forever, and, of course, all of you, my clients, the people I have learned the most from over the years. Thank you for your wisdom, time, love, care, trust, and financial support to help make this book a reality.

This book is dedicated to my Dad.

CONTENTS

PREFACE

"It's no measure of health to be well adjusted to a profoundly sick society." —Krishnamurti

Which basket are you putting your eggs in?

At this moment, I am sitting in a room listening to two people discuss their journey with cancer. Both found out in the last 24 hours that their cancer has progressed. They have both been on their journey for several years.

As I listen to their conversation, I am struck by how consuming cancer is in their lives. They have spent hours, days, weeks, and years doing lab tests, researching, going to doctors, being treated, staying in hospitals to recover from surgeries, and conversing about their fight to survive. Did I mention they are both in their early 40s?

As I sit here listening, I think about the resistance I encounter when I suggest to patients without cancer that they make changes: "I do not have the time... I do not have the money... I do not have the energy." I am sitting here witnessing how much time, energy, and money it takes to fight for your life once you are sick. There is almost no room left for anything else. My heart is breaking.

There are no guarantees in life. However, doesn't it make sense to put your eggs in the basket that supports vitality in your body now? Why not put your time, money, and resources into preventing disease, instead of waiting until you are fighting to survive? After all, isn't prevention your best health insurance?

INTRODUCTION

Every day in America almost every person will, at some point, put something in his or her mouth and swallow it in the act of what we call eating.

After years in private practice observing clients struggle with choices around food, I became curious about what motivates people to eat. I started asking my clients, "Why do you eat?" The responses were illuminating.

Illuminating because I discovered not only why people eat what they eat but also why it didn't matter to them that most of what they were eating wasn't actually food.

Yes, you read that correctly. The fact is that a large majority of what we eat in this country no longer meets the definition of food.

Food: any nutritious substance that people or animals eat or drink, or plants absorb, in order to maintain life and growth.

And this fact is a problem! Based on what I see in my holistic medicine practice every day, it's a really big problem.

What you eat has a direct impact on how you feel today, and how you will feel as you age. And what we are eating is not food.

In the powerful documentary "Super Size Me," Morgan Spurlock spent one month eating only fast food, three meals a day.

Before the month was up, he had completely changed his health **for the worse**; gaining 24 pounds, raising his cholesterol by 65 points, and worst of all, developing a fatty liver.

This happened because he ate the worst form of **C.R.A.P.,** or Chemically Ridden Altered (food) Products. C.R.A.P. is what we are sold to eat that looks like food, tastes like food, but, as you will learn, has little to do with food. And, from my experience, it can make you sick.

In the case of Spurlock's fast food experiment, it only took him three weeks before his health became so impaired his doctor implored him to stop—that's how much damage he had done.

Many of you may be thinking that you do not eat C.R.A.P., and if you do, you certainly do not eat it every day three meals a day like Morgan Spurlock did. The sad fact is, however, that you are most likely falling victim to it more often than you think. C.R.A.P. is hiding everywhere, right in front of your face, even at the best grocery stores.

Almost everything you find in your grocery store has chemicals in it, has been altered from its whole food form, and is now a food product rather than actual food. In other words, it is C.R.A.P. We have forgotten the purpose of food, and we have forgotten that you cannot create health by eating things that are sick and loaded with toxins.

Any race car driver knows never to put low-grade gasoline into his car because he knows it would hinder its performance. Why then do we put low-grade C.R.A.P. into our bodies and expect not to suffer the consequences?

We have lost sight of the fact that if you alter food by changing the soil environment it is grown in, adding in foreign components by fortifying and/or genetically modifying it, as well as introducing chemicals, you are changing that substance.

And if you then eat that product, the changes made are going to affect how you feel and how you perform. Based on how you feel now, how is what you are eating affecting you? Are you vibrant, and full of life, or are you feeling tired? Do you need coffee to jump-start your day? Are you having trouble sleeping, carrying extra weight, in pain, and/or feeling old?

The changes that have been made to food are on your dinner table in the chemically ridden altered food products you are being sold as if they are food and it is affecting your health and your family's health.

The fact is that what you eat matters. It matters a lot! You are literally created from what you eat. Human bodies are not made of chemicals; they are not made of isolated vitamins made in a lab. They are made of nutrient complexes that come from food, air, sunshine, and water.

Early in my practice of using nutrition as a healing tool, a client (we will call Sarah) brought her 13-year-old daughter (we will call Lily) in for care. Sarah reported that the humerus bone in Lily's left arm was deteriorating. It had multiple hairline fractures at the shoulder joint that were causing her pain. She had taken Lily to an orthopedic surgeon and been told that he did not know why this was happening. He also said if it did not heal and continued to progress, the only option would be shoulder replacement surgery. He gave her anti-inflammatory pain medication and suggested she come back in three months for a follow-up. He had no other suggestions.

As you can imagine, both Sarah and Lily were very distressed about the news. Shoulder replacement surgery at age 13, we all agreed, did not sound like a good idea!

I checked her, as will be explained a little later, and found an overload of chlorine in her system.

When I reported this, Sarah's jaw dropped. "She is on the water polo team at school. She is in a chlorinated pool every day," she exclaimed.

"How much chlorine is she exposed to?" I asked.

"A lot," she exclaimed, "...the whole pool area reeks of it."

I paused. I definitely had not learned anything about chlorine and bone deterioration in school, and although I could come up with some plausible theories about how chlorine might be affecting her shoulder, I was anything but certain. I did, however, trust the body. I knew if a body was out of stress and had what it needed, it would heal, so I decided to put aside my "learned knowledge" and trust what I was being shown. There was nothing to lose; supporting Lily's body to more efficiently detoxify chlorine could only be helpful.

I decided to plunge ahead.

I looked at Lily and said, "So exactly how much do you like water polo?"

She looked at me and replied, "It is my favorite thing in the whole world."

Oh boy, now I was in a pickle. Usually avoidance of an offending substance is part of any healing protocol. How could I take away her favorite thing in the whole world?

I took a deep breath, and said to them both, "I am not sure it will work, but rather than making you stop your favorite thing, I suggest we try to clean up your diet and give your body some support in eliminating the chemicals more efficiently and decrease the amount of time you spend in the pool."

After all, there were 30 other kids in the pool with her each day that were not having this problem, so maybe we could help her body not have it as well.

"If it doesn't work," I said, "then we can always have you stay out of the pool entirely for awhile and see if that helps."

They both agreed, glad to have any course of action other than wait and see what happens or, worse yet, prepare for surgery.

We changed her diet from the mostly processed "teenager's diet" she was eating, to one of clean whole food. She was great at making the changes, since her motivation was really high. We added in some whole food supplements to support bone growth and liver detoxification. After the pool, she lathered up with soap to wash away as much chlorine as possible before she turned on the hot shower.

Over the next months, we checked her along the way to make sure her body was improving. Her pain improved, her energy increased, but we wouldn't know for sure if her shoulder was actually healing until her next X-ray.

I remember the day Sarah called me, three months after Lily's initial visit with me. She was so excited, I could barely understand what she was saying. "Wait a minute," I said. "Slow down. What was that?"

She took a deep breath and said, "My daughter's shoulder has healed 100 percent. There are no fractures visible. None!"

Lo and behold, in just a few months, even though she continued to swim and be active, her shoulder had completely healed. It really was a day to celebrate.

Her doctor was so amazed; he thought I was a miracle worker. I wasn't. I had just identified a stress on her body and given it what it needed to handle that stress. Her body did what a body will do if nothing is blocking it —it healed.

What a success story. I was even amazed at the power of good nutrition. But the good news didn't stop there.

Because we had so much success with her daughter, Sarah asked me if I could help her son, Tom. He was not doing well in school and had been diagnosed with Asperger's syndrome, a disorder that can affect an individual's ability to socialize with others and communicate effectively.

She reported that Tom was very literal, and had a difficult time following social cues.

"One day Tom and I were watching TV when someone knocked at the door. He jumped up and ran down the hall to answer the door. I heard a woman's voice ask, 'Hello. Is your mother home?' I heard Tom answer yes and then I heard the door shut. A moment later, Tom was back on the couch. When I inquired to him as to what happened, he reported that she had asked if I was home, he said yes, and then he shut the door and came back to the couch, leaving the woman outside. Having answered her question, he thought the communication was finished."

Today, I could answer questions as to whether nutrition affects brain function without hesitancy. I have witnessed numerous cases of dramatic changes in brain function by improving the nutritional status of a person. However, at that time, I had only been using food as a healing tool for a short while. I had yet to work with anyone with Asperger's, and had no idea if changing Tom's diet could make a difference in his brain function.

So I told her the truth, I didn't really know if I could help Tom with his Asperger's, but suggested she bring him in and see what I could find.

When Tom came in, I noticed he was small for his age. I asked about his diet, and, sure enough, he was eating primarily box cereal and fast food.

I looked directly at Sarah. "Well, I do not know how much we can help with his Asperger's, but I am fairly certain we can improve his health."

We worked together to change his diet from all processed foods to one of low chemical whole foods, like we had done with her daughter. Sarah got rid of all the remaining processed food she had in the house and replaced it with organic whole food. At first, Tom was reluctant, complaining about what he was missing, sneaking fast food when he could.

I kept encouraging him, and, little by little, he made changes.

After a while, he started reporting that he was feeling a little better. "Not sure what it is, but I just overall feel better."

At this point, we discussed his committing to the dietary changes completely for one month. He agreed to give it a try. By the end of the month, when he returned to my office, he reported he was on board 100 percent. "I just feel better eating this way."

About a year later, Sarah came into my office for a check-up. I hadn't heard from her in a while, so I was eager to hear how her children were doing. She looked at me, and tears filled her eyes. "What's happened?" I asked.

She smiled, and I sighed in relief as she went on to say, "I was sitting on the bench behind my son's water polo coaches. I wasn't eavesdropping or anything, just listening a little. One coach started to talk to the other coach about one of the players on the team. He went on and on about how amazing this kid was. What a great player he was and a great leader. It wasn't until the end of their conversation that I realized **he was talking about my son**. It brings tears to my eyes every time I think about it. My son, in just a year, has gone from the awkward bench-warming mascot to someone his coaches think so highly of they have not only made captain of the team, but also rave about to each other in their private conversations."

By the time she was done, I had tears in my eyes and a huge smile on my face as well. Not only was her son excelling at the sport but he was also stepping in as the leader for the whole group.

She went on to say she was completely convinced that the change in his diet made all the difference in her son's life. She had watched as his personality and body changed as he ate real food. The real testament, however, was that he was convinced himself. He felt the difference it made for him as well. He was a true whole food convert.

Since Lily and Tom's success, I have watched repeatedly as my clients have changed their lives using whole food nutrition.

My goal in this book is to help you not only understand but also experience for yourself the difference in how you can feel if you replace the C.R.A.P. you are eating with real honest-to-goodness food. I want you to experience the direct connection between what you eat and how you feel. I want to reacquaint you with how to identify, find, and eat food!

If you are like most people, you are overbusy, overstressed, and overtired. Making a change, no matter how crucial to your well-being, can feel overwhelming and downright impossible.

However, once you grasp and experience how much better you feel, you will understand the only way out of feeling the malaise, the general low-level energy, and the less than optimum wellness is to make a change. And that change includes relearning how to *EAT FOOD!*

In this book, you will read about my "testing" a client, as I mentioned above. What exactly does that mean?

When I am working with a client, I look for areas of the body that are under stress. I do this using a combination of tools: inquiry, lab tests, and a biofeedback system that assesses stress using reflex points grounded in Chinese Medicine. Once an area of stress is identified, I then seek to understand what is contributing to that stress.

Once areas of stress and potential contributing factors are identified, we work to eliminate that stress. Studies have shown that eliminating stress can greatly improve one's health. But nowhere is the evidence more obvious than in the case successes I see in my clinic every day.

I say more than once in this book, "Nothing impacts your health more than the choices you make every day." If you are not feeling well, then I can guarantee you are making choices that are contributing to how you feel.

We are exposed to thousands of chemicals in this country, some estimates say around 85,000. How does your body deal with those chemicals? With nutrients that come from what you eat.

If you are not feeling your best, if you feel like you are aging, if your hormones are out of balance, if you are tired, or if your cholesterol is high, then I can guarantee you that the C.R.A.P. you are eating is playing a role.

I have witnessed so many people change their health by changing the choices they make around food to know with 100 percent certainty that this is true.

This book is not about finding the "perfect" diet. It is not meant to add a new flashy quickly fading diet to the multitudes. The purpose of this book is to inspire you to make nutritional changes for life. It is to remind you of the important role food plays in your health, and teach you how to find and eat real food once again.

I invite you to come on this journey to see for yourself how good you can feel. Commit to following the tenets set forth in this book and you will not only support your own health, but also the health of this planet.

This book is called The Food Solution because by starting this journey you will not only improve your health, you will also become part of a bigger solution. By choosing to eat food, you will be supporting the people who are fighting to make sure real food continues to be available not only now, but also for generations to come. You may think I am kidding, but, unfortunately, I am not. Choose to support your health and you choose to support the entire food chain. That is what I call a win–win choice!

CHAPTER 1

Your Body, Your Choices

Food as the Foundation for Health: My Story

I learned the hard way. At 17 years old, I was diagnosed with irritable bowel syndrome. At the time, there was very little known in the medical community about this condition. In addition, there was no Internet to consult, so no access to the nearly eight million results you get when you do an Internet search on the subject today. So when my doctor told me it was something I would just have to live with, I believed him.

With no medical support, my unhappy belly and I went about living the best we could. In an attempt to feel better, I decided to change the way I ate. I had heard that meat sitting in your intestines turned to poison and since my problem involved a lot of constipation, I stopped eating meat. My doctor had advised me to avoid fiber so I stopped eating raw vegetables and whole grain bread. I felt best when I ate very little, since I always felt bloated and uncomfortable when I did eat. Skipping meals became my best diet plan.

As you can imagine, this was not a sustainable way to live. I was taking in very little nutrition and was extremely thin. However, as a fashion model working in Europe and New York, this seemed like a huge plus! I was in an industry that glorified my rail-thin body, so the fact that no one was giving me a "hard time" about needing to lose weight—as so many of the other girls were getting—was a plus. I just didn't see the problem in my choice.

Mostly, my stomach issue was fairly manageable. My stomach attacks, as I called them, seemed to happen at times when I could deal with them. Except for the time I was at a black tie affair dressed in my most exquisite ball gown and had to beg a ride home in someone's limo because I was in so much pain I couldn't stand up straight.

The real problem was that by not addressing what was going on in my body and eating the way I was eating, or rather **not** eating, I was unknowingly setting the stage for more problems. The combination of poor digestion and poor nutrient intake ultimately led to my body becoming totally depleted. That depletion caused a loss in my body's ability to adapt to stress. So, later in life, when I was exposed to chemicals and black mold, my body had no reserves to meet the increased stress my system was under, and I became ill.

My new health issue wasn't something that came with a diagnosis. I was tired. I was weak. Sometimes, I was so weak I would cry in my car at the thought of having to walk into the house. I went back to the medical world but received little help.

One doctor I saw accused me of having an eating disorder, but never asked me what I ate or why. Another told me I was having low blood sugar episodes, but again never asked what I was eating, or even suggested that I ate. If they had bothered to ask important questions, they would have found out I was eating to manage a problem. I again left their offices thinking I just had to live with it, as I had already been told. Remember, I was in my late teens to early 20s at the time, so my logic was influenced by my youthful exuberance. At this point, I made a conscious decision not to go from doctor to doctor seeking a diagnosis, and continued to "just live with it."

Over time, some of my symptoms improved. My stomach attacks stopped happening, and, although I didn't feel great, I felt okay, and, besides, on the outside, I looked good, so I thought I was okay. What I didn't know was that even though I wasn't in as much pain, my body was still depleted, and my digestive tract still not working well. In other words, on the inside I was still a mess.

Little did I know at the time that it would be my own health challenges that would lead me to the study and practice of natural medicine and the creation of my company, The Sustainable Health Center.

In my late 20s, I decided it was time for a career change, although I had no idea what I wanted to do. I went to the library and checked out books on subjects I liked. One day, I was sitting in the middle of this pile of books looking at the titles when I realized they all had something to do with health. A light went on for me. I wanted to help people with their health (and maybe help myself as well). I knew I did not want to become a medical doctor because, in my own experience, I had received few answers from the medical community for my own health struggles. So, I did a little research and decided to go back to school to study natural medicine. That was the beginning.

In my first nutrition class, I learned that my daily calorie intake was enough to basically "starve" to death. From that point on, I ate three meals a day. Although this helped a little, I continued to be tired and my health continued to decline.

By the time I was in my early 30s, my symptoms were multiple and confounding. Most of them involved pain. I often had the sensation my brain was bouncing up and down in my head when I would wake in the morning. I suffered from bouts of vertigo and always the extreme fatigue that left me exhausted and depressed. I would wake in the morning hurting all over. I constantly felt as if I had a horrible flu, and before I even left the covers in the morning, I would count the hours until I could get back in bed at the end of my day.

But even though I felt really awful, and I mean really awful, I somehow knew I could heal. I knew that taking drugs was not the answer for me. At my very core, I understood that for my own well-being I must learn how my body worked and what it needed to be well.

I spent thousands of dollars seeing natural doctors who prescribed vitamins, and other supplements and I always felt worse when I took them. Nothing I did really helped. Even Chinese medicine, the medicine I was studying, wasn't helping me. Finally, I found an herbalist who was able to keep me out of bed, but no matter how hard I tried, I couldn't get my strength back. I was worn-out to the bone.

It wasn't until I attended a seminar and learned about whole food nutrition—the use of supplements made from concentrated food, as opposed to supplements made from chemicals in a lab, and diet to help the body heal— that things started to turn around for me. I was tested and was given a simple protocol. When I went home, it was like a miracle. I could take everything they gave me and I actually felt the difference.

It turned out that my body had a complexity of things going on. I was very toxic. I had multiple unhealthy bugs in my system, toxic levels of chemicals and heavy metals had built up inside me, and I had developed multiple food intolerances. Simultaneously, I was very depleted and my system was extremely weak. Because of this, I was very sensitive to everything, even treatments.

Whole food nutrition, because it provided the nutrients my body needed to heal itself, was different. Being made from food instead of in a lab—like the vitamins I had tried to take, but was unable to tolerate—made all the difference for me. **Nutrition is what the body uses to detoxify itself, build a healthy immune system, make energy, and rebuild tissue.** Whole food supplements contain the vitamins, minerals, and cofactors as they are found in nature the way a body needs them. So, given what it needed, my body began to do what a body will do if nothing is in its way— heal. I started, for the first time, to feel better, really better. It felt like a miracle. I had found my road toward health.

As my health started to improve, I could really feel when something didn't agree with me. *I was so sensitive.* I noticed the effect of everything. Did it make me feel better or worse? This was when I really started to notice the effect that what I was eating mattered to my health. I started to notice that where I ate, what kind of restaurant, and what I ate really mattered. Slowly, I began to "clean up" my diet and my health improved even more. At this point, I was already in practice and was using diet as one of my healing tools; however, it wasn't until I moved to the Seattle area, and the demographic of my clientele changed that I really saw the powerful difference diet could make.

In Seattle, a large portion of my clientele were raw food vegans. They came in with one health issue or another. I would identify what was going on and support their body, and like most others, they would heal. However, in their cases, it was different. They would heal really fast. This happened so consistently that I began to question why.

In examining them more closely, I found that in general, they had the same life stress as my other clients. They worked a variety of jobs and felt just as satisfied or unsatisfied as the average person feels. The only real difference I could see was their dietary choices.

I looked at their diets carefully and saw that they were 100 percent devoid of processed food. Everything they ate was in its fresh form, organic and free of chemicals. Yes, it was raw, but I didn't think that was the primary factor responsible for their ability to heal quickly, because often I would add cooked food into their diet and their health would improve.

Additionally, any diet that is very one-sided—like a 100 percent raw food diet—can create imbalances and have negative effects on health in the long term, so I wasn't convinced that the food being uncooked was the main reason for what I was witnessing. I started to suspect it had to do with the quality and freshness of what they where eating. When I thought about my own experience of how different things I ate affected how I felt, it all started to make sense. **It isn't what we eat that matters, as much as the quality of what we eat that makes the difference.**

I started playing with my own diet, sourcing and eating only real organic, very clean food. Sure enough, the cleaner the food I ate, the better I felt.

I started to change the focus for my clients as well, making the quality of what they were eating the priority. I encouraged them to source really clean, fresh food.

Just as I had experienced personally, time and again, people who followed my advice and changed their diets towards chemical-free nutritious food felt better, lost weight, and needed my support for shorter periods. There was a direct correlation between them adopting the principles of healthy clean eating and how quickly and completely they healed. Those who fought the changes worked with me longer, required more concentrated food supplements, and needed more frequent office visits.

It has been many years now since I realized this and, to this day, it still holds true. **It is not so much what you eat, as long as you are getting a variety of foods, but rather, more importantly, it is the quality of what you are eating that matters when it comes to your health.**

There are many methods of healing. However, through my years of practice, I have witnessed again and again that no lasting healing will occur without a well-nourished body to support it. You may have an improvement in symptoms. You may even feel better for a while. But if your body does not get what it needs at optimal levels, it will have to compensate. And that compensation will result in a decline in vitality one way or other. If that goes on long enough, the development of a disease of some sort is probable.

This book isn't about the entire healing process; it is about creating the foundation upon which healing occurs. I know with 100 percent certainty that bodies need nutrients to run themselves and to heal. I know with 100 percent certainty that people will not maintain or create optimum health without this foundation.

I know this because I experienced it myself and because I have watched the process over and over again in the countless clients I have helped over the years.

People in this country are getting sicker. Natural health practitioners are seeing it in their clinics at an alarming rate. It is the topic of conversation at all the trainings I attend. What worked once to help people get well doesn't work anymore. We are seeing people get sicker. We are seeing people get sicker younger. We are seeing their illnesses become more and more resistant to treatment.

It doesn't have to be this way. Bodies use food to heal. Give your body healthy, well-sourced food instead of chemicals and you may be surprised at how good you can feel again.

I am finally able to see my illness as the gift it was. But believe me, I didn't always feel that way. Now I know that for me, it presented the opportunity to learn from my own journey. It made it possible for me to help in the healing of hundreds of others in my practice and, ultimately, to share what I learned from those healing journeys with you in this book.

Permanent Change Is the Only Real Way to Solve a Problem.

If you are reading this, then chances are good that you or someone you love is having a health challenge you are hoping to improve. In other words, something inside of you has said you think you can change what is happening. Good for you! Sometimes, admitting to yourself that something needs to change is the hardest step.

If you picked up this book, then you must be suspecting that what you are eating might be playing a role in how you are feeling. Without ever having met you, I can say that I agree. How can I know this about you, a person I have never met? I know this because I have yet to see a person who was not feeling well, whose choices were not part of the problem.

And one choice we make every day is what we put or do not put into our mouth. How can it not be playing a role in how you feel?

I also know it is playing a role because most of what people are putting in their mouth today is problematic. Simply said, our entire food system in this country has a big problem, and that problem is causing us, our bodies, to have a problem.

A problem is defined as:

A matter or situation regarded as unwelcome or harmful and needing to be dealt with and overcome.

So, if there is a problem and we want to solve that problem permanently, we must find a solution. Quick fixes, often medications or fad diets, are not a solution. They are, at best, a short-term respite from the problem.

In order to find a long-term solution, we must admit that what we are currently doing is not working. This is where I often see people start to talk themselves out of what they know in their hearts to be true.

They show up at my office for help. The fact they came is already an indication they know something needs to be done, and they are hoping I will be able to help them affect that change. Yet when confronted with the situation and told changes may be needed, clients often backpedal out of their problem.

They describe to me their current health situation, which we've already established is compromised, but when I offer changes they could make to improve their situation, suddenly whatever it was that got them to me in the first place isn't so bad after all.

This is a very normal human response. Change can feel overwhelming, at times impossible, and often like an enemy we must ward off. But, in reality, change is the only constant on which we can rely. Things are going to change, regardless of our resistance. THE CHOICE OF WHETHER YOU RESIST CHANGE OR EMBRACE IT IS LITERALLY YOURS. The solution is rooted in large part to the choices you make every day. If you make smart, informed, educated, healthy choices, you are going to affect change in a smart healthy way. Do this long enough and you are on your way to a solution. Adjust the way you eat toward cleaner more natural foods and you are guaranteed to raise the level of homeostasis, the metabolic equilibrium, within your body.

I know that changing your relationship to food is the first solution to feeling better not for a little while but forever. Follow my food program for 21 days and you will experience first hand how the food you are eating is contributing to how you feel.

Change is not always easy. I want to start our relationship, just like I do with each of my clients, by being honest with you. You are not going to change your current situation, whatever it is, without making changes in your diet. It isn't going to happen because it just isn't possible. It is against the law of physics. You cannot change how you are feeling today without changing something. And this book is about changing the choices you are making every day around what you put in your mouth.

You Only Get One Body

Are you intensely grateful for your body? If not, you may want to reconsider your position when you remember this one simple fact: YOU ONLY GET ONE BODY!

In this lifetime, you do not get to turn your body in for a sleeker, better model. You do not get to trade it for something stronger, faster, and more resilient. You can make different choices that will strengthen, slim down, or bulk up the body you have, but ultimately you will have some variation of your body, the one you have right now, from now until the end of your time on this planet.

If you were given a car and told, "This is the only car you will ever have, the only car you are ever going to get in your lifetime," wouldn't you take good care of it? What if that car were your only way to get food and water? What if that car were your only connection to the things you love most in your life?

Wouldn't you make sure the oil was changed, the engine tuned, the spark plugs firing, the brakes in working order, all the fluid levels full? Wouldn't you regularly fill it with fuel and wash the windows? Wouldn't you do everything you knew how to do to make it last and be in the best shape it can be for as long as possible? Wouldn't you love and care for it?

Your body is that one and only car you will have. Assume an attitude of gratitude for it. Make choices and decisions that support that feeling of gratitude. Thank your body every day for all it does for you by doing as much as you can for it!

CHAPTER 2

Health and Wellness Basics

"One of the biggest tragedies of human civilization is the precedents of chemical therapy over nutrition. It is a substitution of artificial therapy over natural, of poison over food, in which we are feeding people poisons trying to correct the reactions of starvation." —Royal Lee, 1951

Quick Fixes: You Know It…They *Really* Do Not Work

Too often, in our busy overstressed lives, we opt for the quick fix. We take a pill that makes the symptoms go away. We go on a fad diet or, worse, take pills in an attempt to lose weight. We do a drastic cleanse to rid our bodies of toxins. And we do all this in the name of feeling better.

We tell ourselves things like "I don't have time; I'm too busy or; I'm too tired, too otherwise engaged." Unfortunately, more often than not, quick fixes lead to short-term solutions that not only don't work but also can cause bigger problems down the line.

The seduction is that for a short time, you may experience some relief. You may lose weight from that fad diet or diet pill. Your blood pressure may return to normal as a result of taking a medication. Your acid reflux may disappear from taking that other little pill. Your heartache may go away from ingesting an antidepressant.

But the constitutional reason you gained weight in the first place is not addressed. The imbalance that is causing your body to experience high blood pressure goes unaddressed. The underlying source of your heartburn remains unidentified. The root cause for your depression goes ignored.

And the really sad fact is, as I learned the hard way, that lack of attention in the short term can cost you your health down the road at even deeper levels.

Most prescription medications have negative side effects. You need only watch TV, listen to the radio, or read the accompanying literature to get the litany of horrible consequences common medications can cause. Often, the side effects are worse than the original problem.

For instance, drugs used to treat mild depression are shown to be no more effective than exercise and proper nutrition in treating that depression.[1]

In addition, using some antidepressant type medications can increase the incidence of suicide and violent crime.[2]

Cholesterol medication may lower your cholesterol, but can increase your chances of liver problems and can increase the need for other medications such as Viagra for men, which, in turn, can cause death from sudden cardiac arrest. The medications may lower your cholesterol on a lab test, but you never find out why the body is making more cholesterol, or experiencing an increase in blood pressure in the first place.

Quick fixes may allow you to keep living your life seemingly uninterrupted. But it is a life out of balance and under stress that eventually will catch up with you. A body living under less than ideal conditions will develop further complications. Today those complications are starting to show themselves in younger and younger people.

If you have trouble focusing, are tired, yet amped up, it's most likely not a lack of amphetamines (stimulants) in your body that is causing your problem. It is, however, very likely, as I have seen in hundreds of clients, that your brain isn't getting its optimal blood flow or having its full nutritional needs met.

The lasting, long-term solution to how you're feeling is not a quick fix. It's a lifestyle change. It's the willingness to embrace a new way of thinking, a new way of seeing yourself, a new way of approaching your life and the commitment to making better, healthier choices. Sometimes a quick fix might be helpful to get you over the hump, but do not be fooled into thinking it's a long-term solution because it's not.

Fad Diets: Don't Be a Guinea Pig

Fad: *An intense and widely shared enthusiasm for something, especially one that is short-lived; a craze.*

Diet: *To restrict oneself to small amounts or special kinds of food in order to lose weight.*

There are bookstore shelves lined with books about different types of life-changing diets. One claims the cause of weight gain is carbohydrates. If you avoid carbs and eat only animal products and vegetables, you will never gain weight!

Another claims the root of all illness is animal by-products. If you eat only grains and vegetables, you will be healthy for life!

Another claims the food you eat must be cooked or you will weaken your "digestive fire!"

Yet another claims that unless you eat only raw food, the enzymes needed to properly digest your food will not be present.

And for every diet that exists, there will be someone who swears they have found the one true secret to healthy eating.

The real problem is we are trying things that have never been tried before. In most cases, the latest trend, or a fad diet hasn't really been tried long enough to find out if they are in fact healthy over the long term.

If you look at fad diets or health trends from the past, you can see that what is popular, or the current rage may not always be what is best.

It is obvious now in hindsight that ideas used in the past such as ingesting a tapeworm, or taking up smoking, and/or taking diet pills to lose weight were not good ideas. But at one point, these techniques were all the rage.

Likewise, using mercury to cure syphilis, or replacing breast milk with bottled formula were flat out bad ideas. But do you know that the low-fat diet promoted since the 70s is proving to be bad for your health, and is blamed by many for the skyrocketing of obesity in this country?

I remember when distilled water was the craze, and now, it is recognized that, over time, distilled water leaches minerals from your bones. And, I have already seen the negative effects in my practice of some of the fad diets out there today; extreme cleanses, totally raw diets, and alkaline water.

We don't need to reinvent the wheel. There is nothing new we need to know to support our body's well-being. I know, new is interesting, new is fun, new is sexy, but new is not necessarily better or more effective. As a matter of fact, most of what is being done today that is "new" has contributed to the health crisis we currently face.

Never in the history of man have we seen so many chronic degenerative diseases. Experts say this is due to man's longevity. I wholeheartedly disagree. In "olden days" humans died mostly of exposure to the elements, hard work in adverse conditions, attacks by wild animals, flu, plagues, and bacterial infections.

Today people are dying from heart disease, cancer, the complications of obesity and diabetes, and a myriad of diseases that are degenerative in nature. All these diseases develop over time as a result of our lifestyle choices.

If it were true that our longevity is why we are suffering from these degenerative diseases, then why is it that these diseases are affecting people at increasingly younger ages? Why did I just hear about a 28-year-old mother of two dying from breast cancer just the other day? If it is true that these diseases are on the rise due to a longer lifespan, then why are children developing adult onset diabetes? If it is true, then why are there places on our planet where people live into their hundreds, disease free, and die peacefully of old age in their sleep?

No one can deny we are living longer. But I contend that, if we did a few things differently, we would live even longer and die from old age rather than from degenerative disease. We need only to look at places on the planet where people routinely live productive, vital lives well into their hundreds to see that it is possible. When these places and people have been studied, the one common factor they all share is a diet of clean freshly grown food.

Fad diets and quick fixes will not get you to optimal health. It is true that with certain illnesses, a special diet to help you heal initially may be indicated. A special diet could help you in the short run by drastically shifting the body environment causing pathogenic bugs to die and allowing nutrients that were previously not absorbed to be absorbed. But just because a special diet may help you feel better in the short run, doesn't mean it is a balanced diet that should be adopted for life. Imbalance leads to imbalance.

There is nothing new in this book. All that I write here has been said before. What I share with you are solid principles based on years of clinical practice, not just mine, but a long lineage of whole food health practitioners. These principles were first introduced at the turn of the century when our food first started being altered from its original state. Nothing new, yet, to this day, the ideas are still revolutionary. The majority of Americans are still not aware of the impact that eating processed chemical-laden "foodstuff," as I call it, is having, and they continue to make choices that are making them sick.

To create a strong healthy body, you need nutrients. To avoid developing a disease, you need to decrease your exposure to chemicals. If, at anytime, you should choose to adopt a special diet, make sure whatever special diet you adopt, you still adhere to these principles.

Even with poor nutrition, your body will survive the best it can for as long as it can. Even with an overload of toxins, it is in the programming of your system to survive. Your body will do anything it can to try and be well. But isn't it time to move out of survival mode? Isn't it time to honor your body as the temple it is? Isn't it time to give your body what it needs not just to survive but also to thrive?

Don't be a guinea pig. Make sure whatever new habit you acquire is balanced and has been tested over time. Leave the fad diets behind. Eat nutritious clean food!

Weight Gain, Diabetes, and High Cholesterol: Your Body's Solution to a Problem, not the Problem Themselves!

"If you go on a diet and omit all the fat and eat your starches and carbohydrates that you get in these refined cereals, you will be putting more fat on your back that you can't get rid of. Sugar and flour are the first things to throw out in the diet because they are pure calories and don't contribute anything but fat to the body. —Royal Lee, 1955.

Weight gain, diabetes, and high cholesterol are three of the most common health issues that people face today, and they are more often than not addressed with quick fixes, instead of real solutions. When a health issue arises, the body is often treated as if it is somehow being bad, and nothing could be less true. The body is behaving exactly how it should. It is trying to solve a problem. Instead of supporting the body to heal the problem, quick fixes such as extreme diets, and or medications are given to change the numbers on the scale or lab tests with no thought as to why the body is doing what it is doing.

Let's start by looking at weight gain and diabetes. What is your body trying to do by gaining weight and/or developing diabetes? It is trying to solve the problem of to much glucose (sugar) in the blood or cells at any given moment.

The important qualifier here is "any given moment." Glucose regulation is a very closely monitored system by the body. Too high blood sugar is harmful to your health and will cause tissue damage. This is why diabetics can develop blindness and lose limbs if their blood glucose goes uncontrolled for too long. My father suffered from kidney failure due to standard medical recommendations being unable to get his high glucose levels under control.

But here again is another miraculous function of a healthy body; as a protection, the body will not allow blood sugar levels to remain high, except in the case of diabetes. At any given moment if glucose goes too high, the excess is stored, first in the liver, and, when the liver reserves are full—yep you guessed it—as fat. Consequently, high blood sugar levels are what trigger fat production.

You could fast all day (a bad idea for weight loss by the way) and eat a meal that is low in fat and high in carbohydrates— as is encouraged in many nutrition circles—and you will gain weight. Why? Because whenever your blood sugar level goes too high, your body stores the excess sugar as fat. The carbohydrates are broken down very quickly and the resulting glucose enters your blood stream. Blood sugar that cannot be used is stored, right then and there, in that immediate moment. So you see that weight gain, in most cases, is not because your body is being bad; it is because it is trying to protect itself from too high glucose in the blood. So weight management is really more about blood sugar regulation over the long term than it is about dieting or starving yourself.

Likewise, Type II diabetes is the body's solution to protecting your cells from too much glucose. When high blood sugar levels are uncontrolled for prolonged periods, the cells in the body become insulin resistant.

Insulin is the hormone that carries blood sugar into the cells. When blood sugar levels are high, the body increases the amount of insulin in the blood stream. The high insulin level causes glucose to move out of the bloodstream and into the cells at a rapid rate. To protect themselves, the cells shut down their insulin receptors. They say, "Stop knocking at this door; we are not listening!" All this stems from the beginning problem of too much sugar in the bloodstream. When the situation continues, the cells just stop listening all together and Type II diabetes sets in.

In the case of both Type II diabetes and weight gain, the point is not only how much glucose or calories you are consuming, but just as important is how fast that glucose will hit your blood stream. Simple carbohydrates, as found in processed foods like white flour and added sugar, and even fruit break down very quickly and are moved into the bloodstream at a rapid rate. Complex carbohydrates, like whole grains, starchy vegetables, such as acorn squash or sweet potatoes, legumes, such as kidney and lima beans, break down more slowly and consequently enter the bloodstream more slowly.

Proteins break down and enter the bloodstream even more slowly and fats enter the slowest of all. So from a blood sugar balancing perspective, fat is a very helpful calorie source, since it doesn't cause the rapid rise in blood sugar that processed carbohydrates do.

So, you see, *FAT IS NOT THE BAD GUY!!!* Okay, I know you just threw down your carrot sticks in rebellion—but listen for just a minute. We have made a big mistake in this country and that mistake is at the root of many health issues I see in my clinic every day. We have demonized fat to horrifying effect. Fat, unless eaten in large amounts, does not make you fat. However, added sugar, eaten in small amounts on a regular basis, can contribute to weight gain.

Anyone who has dieted chronically knows that the *calories in, calories out* theory has its limits. You can eat a super low-calorie diet and still not lose weight because the real factor here is how much glucose is in your blood and how much is actually being used in any given moment.

Cholesterol Is Not the Bad Guy Either. Cholesterol is very important to the body. It has many important functions. It is part of every cell membrane. Cholesterol is part of the sheaths that protect nerve cells; it is the beginning material that both your stress hormones and your sex hormones are synthesized from. Cholesterol also plays a role in the synthesis of vitamins like vitamin D. When cholesterol levels rise, it is not because the body is being bad or doing something wrong, it is because the body is trying to solve a problem. That problem could be several different things such as tissue damage due to inflammation, as cholesterol is one way the body repairs damaged tissue, or even chronic stress that is requiring more cholesterol to make stress hormones.

LDL, the supposed "bad" cholesterol, is not cholesterol at all. It is a protein that carries cholesterol away from your liver. HDL, the "good" cholesterol is the protein that carries cholesterol back to your liver to be recycled. The theory is if there is a ratio of no more than 3 cholesterols going away from the liver to 1 going back, then everything is okay. However, LDL increases when more cholesterol is needed—such as when you're under stress and your adrenals need support in making more stress hormones, or when there is tissue damage due to inflammation that needs to be repaired. It is inflammation, not cholesterol, that causes heart disease, by the way.

Taking a pill to lower cholesterol is like blaming the firefighters for the fire and sending them home. Why would anyone do that?

So why are we so obsessed with decreasing cholesterol? Instead, we could choose to look for the problem, the fire.

We may start by changing our diet, minimizing our exposure to C.R.A.P., increasing our nutrient intake, and balancing our blood sugar—as will all happen during the **The 21-Day Diet Detox**— and then assess the state of your health. In many cases, this will fix the problem. If it doesn't, then finding the real cause for your body's need to make more cholesterol is essential.

Please, if cholesterol medication is recommended for you, take the time to find out why your cholesterol is elevated. Remember, medications come with a cost to the body. They have side effects, and they increase the work your liver has to do, increasing stress levels, and, in some cases, even increasing your chance of death. When it comes to diet changes, believe me—avoiding fat and red meat, as is often recommended, is not the solution. Often, the low-est cholesterol I see is in clients who eat a diet high in fat and meat. Cleaning up the quality of fat and meat you eat, as you will read about a little further along, however, may go a long way toward lowering both your stress level and any inflammation in your system.

If cholesterol is a concern for you, you may want to order a cholesterol test just prior to doing the 21-Day Diet Detox and then rerun the test shortly after to see the difference. One client we ran blood tests on had liver enzymes and cholesterol that were so high the lab called me to tell me before I even received the results. I immediately told him to see his doctor. While he waited for his doctor's appointment, he did the 21-Day Diet Detox. When the doctor reran his liver enzymes and cholesterol levels just a few weeks later, they had dramatically improved. This confirmed that his lifestyle choices were part of the problem.

Rather than being mad at your body when it develops a health issue, or punishing it by giving it a chemical with harsh side effects without looking further into why the problem is happening, why not support your body to heal? Start by giving it what it needs to heal itself—nutrition—by increasing the quality of food you eat. Why not lower your stress levels by decreasing your chemical exposure and increasing your activity level? You might just be pleasantly surprised to find out it is not such a bad body after all.

Your Body Has a Secret

Your body has a secret that might be lulling you into believing things are not so bad.

You see, THE BODY IS AMAZING! It can compensate for a lack of what it needs in the most amazing ways. Give it very little and it will find a way to survive as long as it can to the best of its ability.

Symptoms happen when your body is losing its ability to compensate in its current physical environment. Once symptoms manifest, the body is compromised in some way and is doing its best to cope with current conditions.

But why would you want to do that? Why would you challenge your body in that way? Why would you want to just survive, when, with a little conscious thought and a few different choices, you could thrive?

Feeling Old Before Your Time? You Don't Have To

If you think about your future, are you dreaming of a life of pain, dependence on medications, obesity, lethargy, and declining health? I doubt it. However, if you are not making conscious choices about what you eat, where you buy your food, and how you prepare your food, then you may be creating a future that looks just like that without even knowing it.

If you are dreaming of a future full of vibrancy and excellent health where you have all the energy and gusto necessary to manifest your dreams, then taking a step back to assess where you are and what you are doing to support that reality is a great idea.

One area that is really important to assess is what I call our health savings account. How much health savings you have ultimately determines how resilient your system is. Resiliency plays a major role in whether one person recovers from a health issue, say pneumonia, while another doesn't. Resiliency affects how well you will age and how likely you heal when faced with a health challenge.

Over the years, I have watched as people have struggled with the question: "Why me? Why am I sick? Why do I have to eat so pristinely to keep my weight down? Why can my friends eat whatever they want and not have the same problems I have?" Often we feel we are being singled out, punished for some unidentifiable crime. I have to admit, I have felt this way myself at times.

It wasn't until I came across a group of powerful studies conducted between 1932 and 1942 by Francis M. Pottenger, Jr., M.D.[3] that I found the answer to the question, *Why me?* What he discovered was that resiliency has everything to do with what I call your nutritional status and your overall nutritional stores.

Dr. Pottenger was conducting research to develop a new drug, using cats as his subjects. He noticed certain cats had a poor survival rate while others were more resilient. This discrepancy fascinated him and he began to study the cats more closely.

What he found was revolutionary. And, though his work was done some 70+ years ago, his findings are more relevant today than ever before.

Dr. Pottenger discovered what he identified as *third generation cats*, an effect we are now witnessing in our children and ourselves.

When Dr. Pottenger delved into his question about why some cats lived while others died, he found it had everything to do with the food they were eating. And, while this may not have been a shocking discovery—after all, we are what we eat—he realized it was not only the food the cats were currently eating that was determining their resiliency. Equally important was the food their parents ate and, beyond that, the food their grandparents ate.

He found that with each successive generation, the effects of a nutritionally inferior diet were having a greater and greater impact on the health resiliency of the offspring.

By the third generation, cats raised on a nutrient-poor diet, had severely compromised health. Interestingly, they developed many of the chronic degenerative diseases from which Americans now suffer.

Not satisfied with the status quo, Dr. Pottenger went on to see what would happen if he fed fresh, raw food to the nutritionally compromised cats. What he discovered was groundbreaking. Even though the health consequences had been passed down through generations, he was able to reverse these negative effects.

This innovative research is significant for two reasons. One, cats are physiologically very similar to humans. And two, this is the only research done to date that looks at the effects of poor nutrition passed down through generations.

Ultimately, the most exciting aspect of Dr. Pottenger's research is that some of the health challenges we suffer with today may be a result of the diet our parents or even grandparents ate and that this "weakness" **is reversible**.

We are just at the dawn of four generations of Americans eating food that has been altered through processing, and consequently lacking in nutrients.

What generation of Pottenger's cat are you? If your grandparents were farmers, you are probably in better shape than if they were wealthy city folk. That's because wealthy city folk were the ones who could afford the then-cherished canned food, as much a nutritional nightmare then as it is now.

We have only to look at our children to see the devastation of generations of bad eating in the record numbers of degenerative health diseases, diabetes, autism, and other brain imbalances. As for our generation, infertility, Alzheimer's, heart disease, diabetes, cancer, and autoimmune diseases are at record levels.

It is my personal and clinical experience that after generations of eating a nutrient-deficient diet, Americans are experiencing what Dr. Pottenger's cats experienced, a marked decline in resiliency and well-being.

However, there is encouragement from his findings. It took three generations to destroy the health of the cats, but once he added a diet rich in nutrients to the third generation, he was able to reverse the development of disease.

Simply stated, your current health resiliency depends on the health reserves you inherited, and the food choices you have made throughout your life and are making now.

An Economic Model of Health

To explain this further, I like to use an analogy I call the *economics of health*. It is easy for us to understand our monthly financial budgets in terms of being in the black or in the red, in surplus or in deficit. This analogy can make it easier to understand the role that eating plays in your health.

As proven in the Pottenger cat study, we are all born with what I call a health inheritance. How your parents and grandparents ate influences the foundation of your health. As I said, this determines how much resiliency you will have in this life.

As soon as we are born, we begin the process of earning and spending. Earning comes from nutrient intake from food, water, air, sunshine, and love. Spending is a natural part of the biological process that maintains your body. And with each biological function, more nutrients are necessary. The things that determine how much energy you use in a day are dictated by the amount of stress placed on the system.

Biochemically, stress is defined as anything that causes a system to need to adapt. Some of the things that raise our stress levels above biological needs are things that will probably make sense such as the exertion of going for a strenuous hike. However, you may not be aware that exposure to toxins and chemicals; emotional demands, mental demands, unresolved immune challenges, blood sugar swings, and lack of sleep all increase the stress demand placed on your system.

As children in a perfect world, our income of nutrients would be greater than our expenditure. What our body needs on a daily basis to support life would be less than what is available, leaving a healthy surplus of nutrients. This surplus is added to our savings account in the form of muscle, bone, brain cells, nerve fibers, etc. In adulthood, ideally, our nutrient intake and expenditure evens out.

However, more often than not these days, in adulthood, our income, nutrient intake decreases; our expenditures, stress, increase; and we end up in a state of deficit. When we are in the red, so to speak, we have to pull on our inheritance, our health trust fund, to supply the nutrients necessary to keep the body running.

If living in a deficit goes on too long, then our savings start to run out. The body must go into a compensatory mode and budget itself by utilizing available nutrients and energy for core survival. Just as if you had lost a job and would have to budget toward rent and food as opposed to new clothes, your body has to budget toward brain survival, heart health, and acute stress response over other functions, such as skin quality, hormonal balance, the ability to procreate, etc. When there aren't enough nutrients to meet all your body's needs, symptoms start to manifest, and disease can set in.

This manifestation of symptoms is not a sign of your body misbehaving. If anything, it is a sign of your body prioritizing for survival.

To reverse this process in both our children and yourself, it is crucial that you increase the nutrient intake and decrease the overall stress to your system.

Let's use my story as an example. I'm a second **and** third generation Pottenger's cat. In other words, my grandmother was raised on a farm eating farm food and my grandfather was raised in the city eating city food or canned food. My mother was raised eating the standard American diet. I was raised on box cereal, non-fat milk, margarine, bologna sandwiches on white bread, generic brand hydrogenated oil potato chips, and TV dinners. First generation: half nutrient rich/half not. Second generation: nutrient poor. Me: nutrient poor.

Then, when I was eighteen, I was given repeated doses of antibiotics, a huge stress to the system, which led to the development of digestive difficulties.

I was given a diagnosis of irritable bowel syndrome due to stress and told, incorrectly, that I should eat a low fiber diet.

For the next ten years, I lived with improper digestion, which means I wasn't absorbing the nutrients I was eating. Plus I was eating a diet that consisted mostly of processed flour, pasta, tortillas and sourdough bread and, as mentioned before, not eating very much of it.

I had no idea I was on a collision course to illness. I was young. I was successful. I was fit. As a matter of fact, for five years, I was the face of health as I bicycled across America's TV screen as the "Milk Girl." By all standards, I had a great life, yet the combination of my low-health inheritance, a nutrient poor diet, and undiagnosed stressors on my system were depleting my body.

By the time I was thirty-two, my body was done.

Because my health reserves were low in the first place and because I had to spend so much of them rebuilding my body, it has been a much longer process than it could have been, had I known then what I know now. Today I live a very clean life. And my body, although infinitely better, is still rebuilding its reserves.

Because of where I ended up, I am still unable to do things that other people take for granted. I can't have a glass of wine with dinner, eat the "normal" stuff other people eat, such as eggs or most grains, or even over-exert myself without feeling the negative effects, even if it's doing something fun.

Without an abundant health savings account to compensate for the extra draw of energy needed to handle extra stress, my resiliency is still compromised. If I want to feel good, I must live a life that is care-filled and choice-conscious.

If, however, I had learned what I know now earlier and made changes sooner, before my reserves were depleted, I am certain I would have healed much more quickly.

I know this because, in my practice, I watch it happen in others. If we are to heal and live the full productive lives we envision for ourselves, time is of the essence. The further down the depletion road you are, the more difficult recovery becomes. Listen to your body. Tune in to your symptoms. Give your body what it needs. Make sure your savings account is full! This starts with doing something that sounds so obvious and yet requires our attention to fulfill. It starts with eating a balanced, nutrient-dense diet to maintain, and rebuild your stores. And it starts by you choosing to eat food.

END NOTES

1. "Exercise and Depression," last modified June 9, 2009, accessed August 19, 2015, http://www.health.harvard.edu/mind-and-mood/exercise-and-depression-report-excerpt
2. "Suicide & Antidepressants," last modified July 1, 2014, accessed August 19, 2015, http://www.drugwatch.com/ssri/suicide/
3. Francis M. Pottenger, Jr., *Pottenger's Cats: A Study in Nutrition.* (Lemon Grove, CA: Price-Pottenger Nutrition Foundation, Inc., 1983).

CHAPTER 3

Food and Your Body

"One should eat to live, not live to eat."—Benjamin Franklin

Why Your Body Needs Food

Let's start our discussion about the role food plays in your body by looking at your relationship to food.

Sit somewhere quiet, close your eyes, and ask yourself, "Why do I eat?"

Take a minute and jot down your honest answer. Got it?

So what's your answer?

The most common answers I get when I ask my clients are:

"I eat because I'm hungry."
"I eat because I have a craving."
"I eat because I like food."
"I eat because I know I should."

Not one person, not one, answered that they eat to provide their body with what it needs to stay alive and healthy. We have forgotten the *purpose* of eating!

We have forgotten that eating is not solely to satisfy our sense of pleasure or meet an emotional need. We have forgotten that we eat to sustain the growth of new cells, repair damaged tissue, and maintain the vital processes that not only keep us alive, but also maintain our health and vitality. We have forgotten that we eat to not only survive, but also to thrive.

Food, air, water, sunlight, and love are the very foundation from which we sustain life. We eat because nature designed it so that everything we need to survive exists in the animal and/or plant matter we consume, the water we drink, the air we breathe, the sunshine we absorb, and the love we receive.

When I go to a "regular" grocery store, usually to buy sponges, most of what I see that is advertised as edible isn't food! I call it *foodstuff*.

Why isn't it food? It isn't food because it no longer contains essential nutrients. It is no longer made up of unaltered fats, proteins in their natural state, or naturally occurring vitamins and minerals. It no longer contains the necessary elements for your organism, your body, to produce energy, stimulate growth, and maintain life.

How do we know this is true? Look around. The evidence of our malnutrition is everywhere. It is in the declining energy you feel that leads to the need for more and more stimulants. It is in the aches and pains we associate with aging. It is in our PMS and menopausal symptoms that are so prevalent that we think that it is "normal" for women to feel that way. It may be common but it is not normal. It is in our fertility difficulties. It is in the wrinkles in our skin and our low libidos. It is in the dark circles under our children's eyes, in their behavior and learning difficulties.

It is evident everywhere, from your own personal experience to the staggering health statistics devastating this country: one out of two men, and one out of three women is slated to get cancer this year; 29 million Americans suffered with diabetes in 2012; 596,000 people died from heart disease last year.

You can see it in the rise in autism, from 1 in 2000 children in the 1970s and 80s to an estimated 1 in 150 eight-year-olds in the United States today. An increase from 1 in 2000 of any age child to 1 in 150 eight-year-olds is staggering.[1]

It is also evidenced in the autoimmune crisis affecting this country, with an estimate of nearly 50 million suffering today.[2]

But there is good news. This doesn't have to be your future. These statistics can be changed. It's your body. Take back control. The time is now!

Your Role in Your Health

When it comes to the body, we tend to forget we play an important role in our survival. We take for granted that no matter what we do to it, consciously or not, it will keep on keeping on. Our body performs billions of functions every minute that all work toward one outcome—survival.

Survival is the priority of the body. To survive, the heart must beat, supplying oxygen and glucose to the brain. If the brain fails to get oxygen and glucose for even a few minutes, brain cells start to die at a rapid rate. If this goes on too long in the organism, the body will die.

To survive, your body uses resources from the environment. It utilizes oxygen, water, sunlight, and nutrients, and makes energy. It then combines that energy with other nutrients to run organ systems, make new cells, fight off invasions and detoxify or eliminate poisons that would otherwise harm the system.

The body automatically prioritizes whatever serves the next most immediate need. However, we do play a very important role in this process. We supply the body with the water and nutrients it needs by eating and drinking. We supply the necessary raw material. Your body takes nutrients from the food you eat, water you drink and air you breathe, and transforms them into the energy currency of life—adenosine triphosphate (ATP). This high-energy molecule stores the energy we need to do just about everything we do.

If we were to compare our role in the body's survival to the running of a factory, we would be the acquisition department. It is our job to acquire what is needed to run the entire factory. Without our input, all production would eventually cease and since the end product of this factory is survival, we would die.

Unfortunately, most of us have forgotten our role in the successful running of our factory. We lose sight of the importance of what we put in our bodies and what we expect them to do for us in return. We downplay the partnership that exists between our intake and our output. And we turn our backs just when the body needs us to step up and do our part.

Just a Few Things Your Body Does with Food!

Every moment of being alive requires nutrients from the food we eat, the air we breathe, and the water we drink. This being true, how could it be that what we eat does not matter to our health?

When you catch a cold, white blood cells are required to fight that cold. If the nutrients needed to make white blood cells are not available, how can the body make those cells?

If you break a bone and the body doesn't have the nutrients needed to regenerate new bone, how does the body do it? The answer is it doesn't. Or it takes from other tissues, does the best it can, and makes bone that is inferior.

A young girl named Sheila came to my clinic with a broken leg. After months of doing "all the right things," her leg wasn't healing and her doctor was recommending surgery. As I performed body testing on her and asked about her diet, I discovered her body was screaming for protein.

She ate mostly carbs and very little protein, fat, or any other measurable nutrients. I educated her about the importance of protein in bone growth. I gave her supplements to support bone repair and sent her home with clear instructions about how to increase her protein intake. Within two weeks, her leg was completely healed and she avoided a painful surgery.

Although often not as dramatic as avoiding surgery in only two weeks, this kind of scenario crops up in my practice every day. People come in sick, confused about why, and frustrated about how to get well. We teach them how to nourish the body, how to decrease exposure to dangerous toxins. We educate them about the powerful healing machine the body is, if given the proper environment to thrive, and they get better.

Bodies heal. That's what they do…if nothing is keeping them from it. The greatest gift we can give our body is to support it's healing by nourishing it. Don't shortchange your body by ignoring its signals. Your body wants to be well!

The Body is Always Regenerating

The body is constantly regenerating itself. Every few days, cells in the body are being replicated in an ongoing process of keeping you alive.

Replication is the process of one cell producing two new cells. In the body, this results in new tissue being continuously produced. There are varying opinions as to how often this happens, but below are some estimates of how long it takes for various cells in your body to renew.

- Stomach-lining cells - 2 days
- Colon cells - 3-4 days
- Epithelial cells of the small intestine - 1 week or less
- Skin epidermal cells - 2-4 weeks
- Red blood cells - 3 months
- Pancreas cells - 1 year or more

If you have ever been around a person going through chemo-therapy, you may have seen first hand which cells replicate fast-est. Chemotherapy kills off fast replicating cells first. Cancer cells replicate very quickly as do stomach lining cells, hair follicle cells, and certain immune cells. This is why some of the most common symptoms chemotherapy patients experience are hair loss, nausea, and complications from a weakened immune system.

Why do we care that cells replicate? We care that cells repli-cate because they are what your body is made from. Bone, muscle, organs, and all other body tissues are all made from cells. If cells are not replicating then tissue is dying. If tissue is dying, then part of you is dying.

"Two-thirds of a cell is water, which means that two-thirds of your whole body is water. The rest is a mixture of molecules, mainly proteins, lipids (fat) and carbohydrates. Your cells turn the raw materials in the food you eat into the molecules your body needs."[3]

If cells are constantly replicating and repairing your tissue and your cells are made from and constantly using water and nutrients, doesn't it follow logically that in order for them to do their job, they need water and nutrients to complete their mission?

But it doesn't stop there. Cells are made from nutrients. Everything the body does like pumping your heart, digesting your food, or breathing requires nutrients. When the body is getting proper nutrition, it can regenerate itself and heal.

I can't say it enough: the body is a miraculous machine. When we feed it what it needs for well-being, it returns the favor by creating a healthy, vital, organism that can go the distance.

Biotransformation: Keeping Your House (Body) Clean

One of the most important functions of the body, mandatory for survival actually, is biotransformation, commonly referred to as detoxification.

Biotransformation is the chemical alteration of substances such as (but not limited to) nutrients, amino acids, toxins, and drugs. This detoxification is needed to alter nonessential, poisonous, and toxic substances so they can be easily excreted from the body through breath, sweat, urine, and feces.

When we are not eliminating toxins efficiently, either because the body does not have what it needs to run a particular system or because the system is overloaded with too many toxins, the body will eliminate the toxins in whatever way it can. A body that is overloaded with toxins is a body at risk for serious problems.

If a particular system is unable to transform toxins, the body will find another way to eliminate them. Acne is a prime example. As painful as it may be both physically and emotionally, acne is the body's way of solving a problem. In most acne cases, the liver and bowels are overloaded with toxins and unable to function optimally. The body, searching for a solution to an unwanted situation, excretes the excess toxins through the skin. And although acne is not pleasant, I think we can agree it is preferable to having our vital organs, such as the brain or heart, become compromised by an overload of toxins.

When you take hormones or antibiotics as the only solution to solve an acne problem, you may be ignoring the important fact that your system is not detoxifying properly, thus creating a much more serious problem that can lead to other more complex health issues.

We may have biotransformation issues today because the air we breathe, the water we drink, and the "stuff" we eat is loaded with added toxins. We may not be able to control our exposure to the toxins in the air we breathe; however, we can control what is in our food and water. The toxins in our food are a result of the way food is grown, from the way it's handled when harvested, and from the added toxins that are a part of the manufacturing process.

Not only are our bodies being called upon to digest our food, they are also having to do the extra work detoxifying all the added *stuff*. To compound this, when food is processed and chemicals are added, the nutrient density of the food decreases. Essential vitamins, proteins, and oils necessary for detoxification, are destroyed or denatured, robbing the body of its ability to do its job of taking care of itself well.

Transforming and eliminating waste is essential to life itself. Eating *stuff* disguised as food that is loaded with added chemicals only increases the stress on the body. It is vital that we get back to eating real food before we create irreversible damage to the delicate balance of our body's wisdom.

Digestion: The Secret to a Healthy You

You are what you eat, but only if you digest it! In other words, good digestion creates good health; poor digestion creates poor health.

The fact of the matter is: you can eat the best quality food in just the right proportions and balance, but if your digestive tract is not functioning properly, you will not gain the benefit from your good eating habits.

Technically, your digestive tract, which begins at your mouth and extends through the esophagus, stomach, small intestine, large intestine and ultimately to your anus, is considered to be outside your body.

I know. Confusing. *How can it be that these organs, which are clearly inside me, are considered outside me?* The reason is that their contents, until absorbed across a barrier, are separate from your bloodstream and hence are unavailable to the rest of your body.

To move food, i.e., nutrients, from outside your body into your bloodstream and eventually your cells, you must not only eat it, you must also digest it. By that, I mean the food must be broken down into small pieces so it can move across that barrier and into your bloodstream. If this does not happen, you will receive no value from the food and what you eat simply exits your body as waste.

Part of why my health declined so drastically was not only because I wasn't eating a lot of nutrition, it was also because of my digestive problem. I was not absorbing much of what I was eating. Even when I did increase my food intake, my health only improved a little.

The act of digesting food is quite complex, involving multiple stages and many substances. However, since this information could literally save your health, I am going to share with you the highlights of that process, just the bits that will help you make informed choices, making the information—and your food—easier to… "digest."

As soon as you put food in your mouth and begin chewing, digestive enzymes are released in the form of saliva. These enzymes are necessary to separate individual nutrients from complex animal or plant material and break them down into their primary blocks to support absorption. No chewing and/or no salivary digestive enzymes impairs absorption. It's that simple.

The salivary enzymes begin the digestion of carbohydrates and fat and act as the first line of defense for your immune system. When you swallow your food, it travels to the stomach via the esophagus. Once food reaches the stomach more enzymes plus hydrochloric acid (HCl) are released.

HCL is responsible for creating the necessary acidic environment for proper protein and mineral absorption to occur. Low HCl levels, which translates as too high a pH (the measure of acid levels) in the stomach, creates an environment where the enzymes will not function properly. This results in protein and minerals not being broken down and absorbed, and it can be a main cause of diseases such as anemia and osteoporosis as well as contributing to a multitude of other health issues, as you will see.

When the food mixes with enzymes, it forms what is called chyme. The chyme is then released from your stomach into the small intestine at a pH of 1 to 2, very acidic.

Once the chyme is in the small intestine, where most of the nutrients that have been broken down are absorbed, the low pH stimulates the release of more enzymes as well as bile from the gallbladder and bicarbonate from the pancreas. These substances play a vital role in proper digestion.

Bile and bicarbonate are very alkaline and they combine in the small intestine to counter the acidic level of the chyme, bringing it to a more neutral PH that the small intestine enzymes require for optimal function.

Bile supports the breakdown of fats, playing an essential role in the absorption of vitamins A, D, E, and K: all the fat-soluble vitamins. The pancreatic enzymes continue the breakdown of carbohydrates, proteins, and other matter, such as phytonutrients found in food.

Bile also serves an important function in detoxification. In the process of making bile, the liver adds in toxic substances to be removed out of the body. When bile is released, these substances are carried out of the body into the digestive tract for elimination through the stool.

It's a busy world inside that body of yours and we're not done yet.

As the chyme passes from the small intestine toward the large intestine, in a healthy digestive system, only those substances that have broken down into a manageable size are able to make it through the intestinal wall and into the bloodstream. Once the chyme reaches the large intestine, bacteria breaks down the proteins and starches that were not fully digested. When all of the nutrients available have been absorbed, water is reabsorbed from the chyme and the remaining waste material is expelled from the body.

In the large intestine, water and electrolytes are reabsorbed, making the stool a soft well-formed consistency. If any part in this cascade is missing, digestion can be negatively affected.

Remember, all of this activity is dependent on the stomach being the right pH, hence on HCl being present. It is essential for not only the proper breakdown of nutrients but also the stimulation of peristalsis (the movement of muscles in the digestive tract that promote bowel movements), the release of enzymes, and creating the right environment for a healthy gut flora.

HCl is the king when it comes to digestion. And, in this country, we blame it for everything from heartburn to coughs and even fake heart attacks, and hence set out to eradicate it from existence. It's become a $10 billion a year acid-blocking business.

The Universe Within

Within the stomach, the digestive tube is a universe of microorganisms, also known as gut flora. Bugs, I like to call them. There are literally trillions of these very important bugs in your body. I know what you're thinking: *What would I want with trillions of bugs?* But the truth is, these bugs literally keep you alive and they rely on the correct environment (i.e., pH) to survive.

Our bodies live in a very symbiotic relationship with the bugs as their life cycle produces byproducts that help us survive. They play a role in everything: the making of vitamins, breaking down of food for absorption, and even the alerting of our immune system to the presence of harmful substances.

Research shows that these bugs can trigger or prevent disease, influence our moods, and in animal studies, have been proven to have a direct effect on behavior.

As far as our end of the bargain, we play the perfect host by supplying these bugs with all the right *stuff* for them to survive. We even determine the kinds of bugs that will thrive depending on the environment we provide.

When we are under a lot of stress or our system is exposed to processed foods, high sugar intake, antibiotics, chemicals, heavy metals, or unresolved emotional traumas, the environment in our intestines changes. With this environmental change comes a change in the types of bugs that take up residence. Often the new bugs are not symbiotic with our systems but rather opportunistic.

They produce byproducts that are toxic to our system, robbing us of vital nourishment and creating an environment that requires our body to do more work to eliminate the toxins they produce.

In other words, they become a drain to our body, increasing its stress. This can lead to dysbiosis, a state of imbalance of good and bad bugs in the body that can often result in illness. As a matter of fact, an estimated, 98% of people I've worked with over the years have been suffering with some form of dysbiosis, many of them not even aware they have digestive problems at all.

Let me take a moment here to discuss a rather important function of digestion, the digestion of fats. The digestion of fats is paramount to our health across many areas. One area you may be hearing a lot about these days is brain function. Without enough healthy fat, brain function does not happen at optimal levels and could lead to brain degeneration. Much of the research being done today is confirming what whole food nutrition based practitioners have known for years; low fat diets are harmful to your health and particularly to the health of your brain.

Correcting your diet is the first step to creating a healthy environment for good bugs to thrive, and for your digestive system to do its best work. Most of us realize that how often we eliminate is a good barometer of our digestive health. However, you may not realize that you could be having a bowel movement every day like clockwork and still be suffering from an unidentified bowel issue. If you experience bloating, gas, irregular bowel movements, (less than one per day and no more than three to four a day) and your bowel habits do not change with dietary changes alone, further investigation is needed.

But don't look to your gut alone to determine if your digestion is functioning properly. Did you know that if you have congested sinuses, pain anywhere, especially in your back and joints, allergies, seasonal or otherwise, acne, or even arthritis, those symptoms are also a sign that digestive issues could be contributing to the state of your health?

Here are the simple facts. You will not change your digestive issues if you do not change your eating habits. And you will not correct your health issues until you get your digestion function in proper working order.

Acid Reflux

Not only is acid reflux one of the most misunderstood health issues in America, but the treatment most commonly prescribed is one of the most dangerous.

In order to break down protein, absorb minerals, and make vitamin B12, hydrochloric acid (HCl) must be present. The stomach must be in a very acidic state to prepare chyme, food that has been partially digested before being released into the small intestine. If HCl is not present in a high enough quantity as often happens as we age or when we are under stress, the release of chyme from the stomach into the small intestine is delayed. This delay causes food to rot in the stomach. That rotting leads to the production of acid that eats away at the stomach and is experienced as burning. If you experience burning a few hours after eating, you can rest assured that this is what is happening in your stomach.

When you take an acid-blocking medication, the commonly prescribed daily pill, you feel better because the overall acid level is lower. However, now you have masked the symptom and are no closer to solving the core issue that is causing the burning. In addition, by artificially creating a lower acid level, you have created other potential problems because now your mineral and protein absorption is impaired, which can contribute to anemia and/or low calcium levels.

When my grandmother was told she had the beginnings of osteoporosis, her doctor recommended that she consume a common over-the-counter antacid medication that was high in calcium to increase her calcium levels. When she relayed this to me, I was not pleased. I tried to explain to her why this was not a good idea.

First of all, in order to absorb calcium, a certain level of acid is necessary in the stomach and secondly, the calcium used in the over-the-counter antacid is a form that is not absorbable. I also explained that when the acid level is low, the absorption of other minerals such as iron would be impaired, not to mention that calcium, in and of itself, blocks iron absorption.

Unfortunately, because the recommendation came from her doctor, she continued with his suggested course of treatment. It wasn't until her health started to decline and she developed anemia that she began to think I might have been on to something.

If you take HCl supplements and feel worse (i.e., experience more burning), this could be an indication that your stomach lining has been damaged. Once the stomach lining has eroded, acid—no matter what the quantity—will cause burning. And the digestive lining must be restored to health before HCl can be taken. If you are at this point, then you can be sure you have an unhappy digestive tract and you should seek the support of a licensed healthcare provider.

A couple of other causes of acid reflux I commonly see are food intolerances or a fungal overgrowth that irritates the lining. In these cases, the source of the inflammation must be eliminated: the food causing the irritation must be avoided, and the fungal overgrowth healed before there can be any relief from the burning.

Another dangerous side effect of low levels of HCL is the potential for vitamin B12 deficiency, which can cause a myriad of health problems. One of the most life-threatening issues is the direct correlation between low levels of vitamin B12 and high homocysteine levels. Elevated homocysteine is considered one of the best predictors for the development of heart disease.

Over the years, I have seen more people with mineral deficiency, due to the use of acid-blocking medications than any other kind of deficiency. In my opinion, taking acid blockers as a long-term solution for acid reflux is one of the most dangerous Band-Aids used by the medical profession. There is nothing that will deteriorate your health more over time.

Likewise, taking digestive enzymes or hydrochloric acid long term, in most cases, are not optimal solutions either. A body working at its optimum should be able to manufacture its own enzymes. Having said that, periodic enzyme support to normalize digestive function, especially under times of digestive imbalance or high stress, can be helpful. Just be sure they don't become a way of life. Check with your healthcare advisor to see if digestive enzymes could help you improve your health.

Stress and Your Health

The human body is designed to experience stress and react to it. When we think of stress, we commonly think of what is known as fight or flight. However, that is just a small portion of the stress response in the body. The stress response includes many reactions in the body. Basically, when the body has to make a change to adjust to the environment, a stress response is elicited. Stress is a normal healthy part of living.

A well-functioning adrenal system, the system that manages our stress response, helps us adjust to the twists and turns that come our way on a daily basis. When your adrenal system is over-taxed, a condition I experienced during my illness, the body loses its ability to adapt to the environment.

A myriad of things can happen when we lose our ability to adapt. Tolerance for other people declines. Our hearing can become more sensitive, making even small noises irritating. Sleep can become difficult; we can lose our ability to handle missing a meal even for a short period. Even our ability to handle things that would normally elicit a feeling of joy, such as children playing, can be difficult.

A stress response may be triggered from external sources; a car suddenly pulls out in front of you or a colleague at work is being difficult. Or it can be generated from internal sources; toxins accumulating in the body in the form of heavy metals, untreated infections, too much sugar, or even your thoughts.

Minimizing stress when you can is always a good idea. But eliminating stress altogether is not only impossible, it's actually not even desirable. Your body's ability to respond and adapt to stress is a sign of good health.

However, stress that goes unresolved for long periods can create what is called "dis-stress," and invariably results in negative consequences to your health.

A continuous barrage of challenges can bring stress to dangerous levels. When we feel trapped by our circumstances and are unable to get relief, we are on our way to stress producing negative effects on our health. When this happens, we have moved out of a healthy stress response and into a state of distress.

If you have trouble falling asleep more nights than not, or you regularly wake in the middle of the night because your mind won't stop, you may already be in a state of distress.

The stress response is moderated by several hormones; the two most important are adrenaline and cortisol.

Adrenaline increases your heart rate, elevates your blood pressure, and boosts energy supplies. This was designed so you can get away from that tiger that is about to attack you. Cortisol, the primary hormone that helps us adapt to the stress of daily life, increases sugars (glucose) in the bloodstream, enhances your brain's use of glucose, and increases the availability of substances that repair tissues. Once you've escaped the tiger, now you want to relax. Both hormones are made from nutrients in the food we eat.

Stress hormones are designed to help the body survive in the immediate moment. So when stress hormones rise, nonessential functions like the immune response, digestion, and sex hormone levels go down. Let's face it; if you are being chased by a tiger, getting away is much more important than getting pregnant. If the stress response is stuck in the "on" position, as in the case with chronic distress, then the function of the immune and digestive systems, the reproductive system, as well as the regeneration of certain tissue and cells, will decline.

Take a body that is in a state of poor nutrition, add ongoing unrelenting stress, and you can end up with low stress hormone levels that can seriously compromise your overall health, let alone the quality of life.

Once your body's ability to adapt to stress has been compromised, the road back to good health can be slow, arduous, and frustrating.

John came in to see me. He was really excited. He was in recovery from a long history of alcohol use and was making great strides in changing his life. He felt pretty good overall, but just wanted to make sure everything was okay. From outward appearances, he looked healthy. He had already lost lots of weight, had made great changes to his diet, and was really committed to changing his emotional relationship to his life. In other words, he was on a solid road to recovery.

Although he felt good, I was a little curious about what I would find. Obviously, with his history, his body had been under a lot of stress for a long time. Yes, he felt good, but was he really feeling good or was his "good" just a comparison to how he used to feel?

As we started to work together, I saw a pattern emerge. One week he'd feel pretty good, the next he would have trouble getting out of bed. I noticed he crashed anytime he encountered extra stress. So, I suggested we run some labs to look at his adrenal health. I had begun to suspect low cortisol reserves were part of the problem. Sure enough, when I got his lab results his cortisol reserves were very low. He was not able to cope with any additional stress, whether it was the stress placed on his system from some emotional incident, or whether it was stress placed on his system from catching a cold.

Once we identified this, we were able to adjust his program to accommodate for these low reserves and support him in making changes that would ultimately help him restore them.

Although not everyone is going to have this level of low reserves, I do see distress playing a major role in almost every person I work with. As a matter of fact, I am willing to say I see distress as the underlying cause of most people's health issues.

Because cortisol decreases the immune function, one sure sign that a body is under too much chronic stress is when a client says to me, "I never get sick." Never getting sick is not normal, nor is it healthy. A good old-fashioned cold once in a while is a sign that your system is up and working properly. Since stress hormones suppress the immune system, when someone is never getting sick, it is very likely I will find a host of unresolved immune challenges in their system, bugs that have been able to go undetected by the suppressed immune system.

Internal vs. External Stress

Most people think of stress as being caused by something outside themselves: you have a deadline looming you feel you can't meet, you miss your flight, or you are stuck in traffic on your way to an important meeting. All of these factors can definitely cause stress.

But our bodies know how to combat these fight-or-flight scenarios. We are physiologically prepared for this kind of stress. We know how to cope because our bodies can manage a fleeting stressful situation.

But there is a silent, potentially life-threatening stress that we may never realize we are harboring until it is too late. That is the internal stress, which, over time, drains our system, uses up our nutrients, and can lead to an overall physical decline. The most common internal stressors I witness in my practice are:

- Unresolved infections or other immune system imbalances (as mentioned above)
- Chemical or heavy metal build-up
- Food intolerances
- Nutritional deficiencies
- Blood sugar swings

And to add insult to injury, when the body is under stress on the inside, our ability to handle the ebbs and flows of life decreases, making our response to our external environment feel more stressful. We get caught in a vicious cycle and, over time, this chronic dilemma can lead to other problems such as low adrenal function, inflammation, and poor detoxification.

Initially, stress hormones are high, which has the effect of not only suppressing the immune system, but also slowing down healing and repair, destroying healthy muscle and bone, coopting biochemicals needed to make other hormones such as the sex hormones estrogen and testosterone, impairing digestion, wreaking havoc on mental function and affecting our ability to fall asleep. If this goes on long enough, your ability to make stress hormones can become impaired, leading to low hormone levels.

Once you have low stress hormone reserves, life experiences that were once no big deal can start to feel like insurmountable affairs. So once reserves are low, the low reserves themselves increase your experience of stress, which only worsens the problem.

Also, when adrenal reserves are low, inflammation sets in. Pain levels can increase since cortisol plays a critical role in helping the body to moderate inflammation, and detoxification becomes hindered. Once detoxification is hindered, tissues in the body become exposed to harmful substances in higher amounts and for longer periods. This of course increases inflammation, creating a body that is in pain, overloaded with toxins, and under a huge amount of stress.

It is nearly impossible to decrease the experience of external stress when there is a high level of internal stress. The body simply does not have the capacity to handle everyday stress when the overall system is already taxed by an ever-present internal stress.

Take the case of Ray, a reluctant client who had reached his wits end and came to me in search of answers.

"I don't get it. I've got a steady job with the government. I mean, you don't get more secure than that in these times, right?" Ray started.

"Well, it is important to feel a sense of security, sure." I replied. "What else is going on?"

"I don't know. I'm just… depressed, I guess. I don't know. And anxious. I feel anxious all the time. I really hate working in the cubicle at work. I do not know what to do, I can't afford to change jobs, but I just hate it. Every time I walk in the door, I start to feel anxious. And now, well, the most disturbing thing…"

He paused and I knew the real motivator for why he came to see me was about to be revealed. I looked straight at him and with my most encouraging smile said, "It's okay, Ray. The more information you share with me, the better I can help you make a difference in your life."

"Things aren't, you know… working down there as good as they used to," he said, looking at his shoes.

And there it was, the "big fish." For many of us, when it comes to our health, we seem to have a pretty high tolerance. We can accept feeling just okay, even occasionally pretty bad, because we think that it's normal, or temporary. We don't realize how good we can feel if we make the conscious choice to give our bodies what they need to function optimally.

Ray was finally experiencing a symptom he couldn't live with. He had come to accept depression and anxiety as normal. And, as so often happens, it took an important function or dysfunction of his body, to get his attention.

In our work together, we assessed his body and identified areas of internal stress. Over the next several weeks, I introduced him to a new way of looking at food. And he began to make dietary changes. I identified and helped him eliminate an immune challenge in his intestines. We also did some emotional clearing around his work. In other words, we did several things to decrease his internal stress level.

"I can't tell you how much better I feel," he reported one day. "My anxiety has decreased tremendously and I'm not at all depressed. It's a miracle."

"And that other issue?" I inquired gingerly.

He smiled. "Oh yeah. I'm all good on that, too!"

"That is great news!"

"Oh, and the other thing," he started.

"There's MORE?" I said laughing.

"I know, hard to top that, but yeah, there's more."

By this time, he was laughing too. Continuing his story, he said, "One day last week I got the idea to take pictures of the sites my department is working on. I just did it on my own time but I thought that maybe they might like the idea and since I love doing it, it seemed like a no-brainer."

"Good for you!" I said.

Once his internal level of stress had decreased, he was able to look anew at the problem that before felt completely unsolvable. One of the side effects of feeling good is that we are open to new ideas, inspirations that simply can't come to us when our bodies are shut down or not working at their highest level.

Ray went on. "Thanks! But the best part is, I showed them to my boss and he loved the idea of having visual representations of the projects we're working on and suggested I continue taking them."

By now, I was grinning ear to ear.

"He gave me permission to go out in the field during regular work hours and take photos. I mean, it's not my dream job, but compared to where I was a few months ago, I feel like anything is possible!"

This is a prime example of how decreasing internal stress can lead us to look at our external environment and find solutions that did not even exist before in our consciousness.

And the first step to alleviating internal stress is making the necessary dietary changes. When we supply our bodies with a variety of clean nutrient-rich food, and we decrease our exposure to chemicals, we supply the body with the support it needs to handle the immune challenges, toxins, and other internal factors that are increasing our internal stress level. When our internal stress goes down, our ability to handle and find solutions to the situations in life that feel stressful improves.

By following the 21-Day Diet Detox, you will be taking the first step towards doing exactly that. The Diet Detox was designed to help you get the C.R.A.P. out of your diet and by doing so decrease the level of your internal stress. In just 21 days, you will create an environment that decreases inflammation, and supports healing in your body.

For some people, doing the 21-Day Diet Detox and then implementing the dietary changes outlined in this book on a permanent basis will be all it takes to really turn your internal stress off. For others, the dietary changes will be the first step in your healing journey. But regardless, making the dietary changes outlined here will decrease the internal stress being placed on your body by the C.R.A.P. that is currently sneaking into your diet and create the environment for your body to heal.

END NOTES

1. "Kathleen Doheny, "Autism Cases on the Rise; Reason for Increase a Mystery, WebMD, accessed August 23, 2015, http://www.webmd.com/brain/autism/searching-for-answers/autism-rise
2. "Autoimmune Disease Fact Sheet," accessed August 23, 2015, http://www.aarda.org/autoimmune-information/autoimmune-statistics/
3. "What Is a Cell Made Of?" accessed August 23, 2015, http://www.sciencemuseum.org.uk/whoami/findoutmore/yourbody/whatdoyourcellsdo/whatisacellmadeof.aspx

CHAPTER 4

The Changing Nature of Food

"We have drifted into this deplorable position of national malnutrition quite inadvertently. It is the result of scientific research with the objective of finding the best ways to create foods that are non-perishable that can be made by mass production methods in central factories, and distributed so cheaply that they can sweep all local competition from the market. Then, after there develops a suspicion that these 'foods' are inadequate to support life, modern advertising steps in to propagandize the people into believing that there is nothing wrong with them, that they are products of scientific research intended to afford a food that is the last word in nutritive value, and the confused public is totally unable to arrive at any conclusion of fact, and continues to blindly buy the rubbish that is killing them off years ahead of their time."—Royal Lee, Founder of Standard Process, June, 1943

A Brief History of Food

Food: Edible or potable substance (usually of animal or plant origin), consisting of nourishing and nutritive components such as carbohydrates, fats, proteins, essential mineral and vitamins, which

... sustains life, generates energy, and provides growth, maintenance, and health of the body.[1]

So, for something to be considered food, it must do several things. It must be able to sustain life, help us generate energy, and promote growth, which I think we would all agree the stuff we are eating is doing to some degree. However, it also must be full of nutrition, and it must support the body to be healthy.

The fact is that, most of what is sold in supermarkets, at fast food restaurants, at chain restaurants, at liquor stores, and even in some health food stores, no longer meets this definition. It no longer contains enough nutrition to do this. This is why even though it may look good, it is now more C.R.A.P. than it is food.

Let's start by taking a look at what has gone missing from your food that is contributing to this being true.

If you sat down to the same dinner your grandparents enjoyed 100 years ago, you would not begin to get the same level of nutrition they did. Why? Because the way we grow, harvest, store, ship, and process food has changed so much that our food and, subsequently, your health is suffering the consequence of these changes. And that consequence is unfortunately, an inferior altered product that no longer contains the naturally occurring nutrients that your body needs to stay healthy.

Right after World War II, we dramatically altered the fertilizer we use in this country. The U.S. government had built several new factories to supply nitrogen for bombs, and after the war, they needed them to serve some purpose and they were converted to produce ammonia-based fertilizer. By, 1981, in the United States, the use of organic fertilizers, derived from plant and animal matter, had been replaced by chemical fertilizers to the tune of 24 million tons per year.[2]

That means 24 million tons of chemicals and inorganic minerals have been added to your food instead of nutrient-rich organic fertilizers. At first, this seemed like a great thing as chemical fertilizers do increase crop yield. However, we now know that they have the unfortunate added effect of destroying soil quality and decreasing the nutrient density of the end product—our food.

According to the U.S. Department of Agriculture, inorganic fertilizers usually contain only a few nutrients—generally, nitrogen, phosphorus, potassium, and some sulfur, the primary nutrients plants use to grow. Because these nutrients are in a concentrated form in inorganic (chemical) fertilizers, readily available to plants, plants grow quickly. However, the nutrients in chemical fertilizer, listed above, are only a limited few that the human body needs to thrive. So when chemical fertilizers are used, as in all commercial farming today, the byproduct is food that is inferior in quality because it is lacking in nutrients that would be there if natural fertilizer were used.

In addition to speeding up the growth process of plants, these fertilizers also support the rapid growth of weeds. To solve the weed problem, chemical glyphosates, found in the common herbicide Round-up, are used to thwart weed growth. Add in the need to genetically modify the seeds to resist the glyphosates, and you have a double whammy that combines to decrease the quality of what you buy at the supermarket.

In recent studies, these glyphosates have been shown to kill off healthy microorganisms in the soil and promote the growth of unhealthy fungi.[3]

The microorganisms in soil play an essential role by breaking down naturally occurring plant matter into vital nutrients and aiding in the absorption of vitamins and minerals not otherwise found in the chemical fertilizer. Without this natural process, soil is converted from a rich dark loam loaded with nutrients, into a pale lifeless substance.

These farming techniques are being blamed for the loss of 65% of the topsoil in this country. That is a staggering number. Without topsoil, food cannot grow. And once the topsoil is killed, it does not come back. It blows away and erodes, and the land where it was eventually becomes a desert.

These practices are used on a large scale in non-organic commercial farming, thus compromising the nutrient density of what you are eating. According to the report, *Still No Free Lunch,* "Food scientists have compared the nutritional levels of modern crops with historic, and generally lower-yielding, ones. Today's food produces 10% to 25% less iron, zinc, protein, calcium, vitamin C, and other nutrients, the studies show."[4]

Because the crops are grown in this sub-optimal soil, the plants become very prone to pest infections, making the need for pest control increase dramatically. Increased pests, increased use of pesticides to the tune of over 1 billion pounds of pesticides are used in the United States each year.[5]

I could write a whole book about the negative effects of pesticides on your health, but for simplicity's sake, let's just quote the Environmental Protection Agency's own website. "The health effects of pesticides depend on the type of pesticide. Some affect the nervous system. Others may irritate the skin or eyes. Some pesticides may be <u>carcinogens</u> (cause cancer). Others may affect the hormone or <u>endocrine</u> system in the body."[6]

This makes them a potential link to breast cancer that, in my opinion, cannot be ignored. Pesticides have been shown to affect the developing brain in children.[7]

Standard commercial farming practices are to pick vegetables and fruits before they are ripe. Have you ever wondered why tomatoes bought at the store taste like waxy cardboard? I was recently having a conversation with the owner of the local organic food delivery service in my neighborhood, talking about food, one of my favorite subjects. He told me about a shipment of peaches he had received the previous week.

"They were hard as rocks," he exclaimed. "Unfit for human consumption!" When he called the supplier to see what was going on, they sheepishly apologized and said he had accidentally gotten a shipment of fruit intended for one of the large health food store chains and promised to correct the mix up. They knew he would never sell fruit picked unripe to his customers. Why? Because a fruit picked before it's ripe is vastly inferior to a naturally ripened one.

The longer a vegetable or fruit is attached to the plant, the more time it has to absorb all the good things in the soil. Picked too early, it lacks much of the nutrition it would otherwise contain. Not to mention it is sorely lacking in flavor!

The sad truth is, the practice of using chemical fertilizers, pesticides, and picking while still unripe is driven purely by economics, certainly not by your health or taste buds.

Often these fruits and vegetables are grown in some far away country, sprayed with a chemical to halt ripening, shipped thousands of miles to a warehouse where they sit until the price point is right to sell. Then they are sprayed with another chemical to promote ripening. In other words, all this is done to make them soften and turn the right color for consumer comfort. Be assured that not one of these processes has anything to do with offering more nutrients.

As consumers, we must take some responsibility for our role in this process. We have a certain expectation of how we want our fruits and vegetables to look. If they aren't picture perfect, we loathe buying them. And it's how we spend our money that determines how stores conduct their business. So, if we won't buy them unless they're blemish free, they aren't going to put the less than perfect produce on display. If it suddenly became cool to buy imperfect fruit or veggies, I can guarantee they would start selling them.

I was at the farmers market one day, and an elderly lady was picking through the corn very carefully. I was fascinated.

"Excuse me," I said. "May I ask what you're looking for?"

"I'm looking for the corn with the worms on them. The worms are smart; they know which ones are good."

I have to say I'm not sure I would choose my vegetables by that same method, but the contrast to our current blemish-averse choices, certainly put a smile on my face. And it let me know that the corn was indeed organic and free of pesticides.

The challenge for the average consumer is that it is almost impossible to know whether the whole foods we buy are nutrient-dense and clean or nutrient lacking and filled with chemicals. It is impossible to tell because commercial food production is expert at providing great-looking food products.

All these practices serve to bring you cheaper produce, to the benefit of the manufacturer and the perceived low cost benefit to the consumer. But is the low cost really a benefit to us?

The average person in the United States spends a lower percentage of income on food than people in most other countries spend.[8]

Yet the USA spends more money on healthcare than any other country.[9]

Now spending more on healthcare would be fine if we were healthier than people in other countries were. Unfortunately, we are not. U.S. health markers are not only rated as being low as compared to other countries, but also they are getting worse. We have dropped to the 27th spot out of 34 countries in terms of early deaths from 1990 to 2010. Meanwhile, our healthy life expectancy fell from 14th to the 26th ranking.[10]

So yes, we are spending less of our income on food than other countries, but we are also spending more on healthcare and our rankings on key health statistics are dropping dramatically as compared to other countries.

Since what you eat plays such a major role in your health, perhaps this cheap food we are buying is actually coming with a very high price tag attached to it. And I don't mean just the dollar price attached to our higher healthcare costs but also the expense of your invaluable, irreplaceable health.

Turning Food into C.R.A.P.!

So now, we have these fruits, veggies, grains, and legumes that are already lower in nutrition, and then we process them. Processing is the practice of altering food from its original form, again usually with the goal of making it more appealing to the customer, and increasing its shelf life. The evidence that processed food is drastically lacking in nutrition is clear.

How do you think the process of fortifying food came about? Food is fortified because, when processed, the nutrients have either been removed or destroyed. If they tried to sell their products in this condition, nutritional deficiencies would become rampant, as happened years ago when food first started to be altered from its natural state.

Have you ever wondered why milk, a food known to be high in vitamin D has vitamin D added to it. It's because it was destroyed during pasteurization. Have you ever stopped to wonder if anything else was destroyed? The answer is yes by the way, but are you certain everything that has been removed has been replaced? What else are you not getting?

What about the nutrients in meat? Do the chemicals and fillers added to meat prior to selling alter the nutrition? I know when I stopped eating commercially raised and processed meat and replaced it with minimally processed, cleaner, more humanely raised meat my health improved. Is it because I am no longer consuming the chemicals or is it because I am now getting more nutrition? I honestly can't say. All I know is my health improved.

Ever since I learned in the movie *Food Inc.* that meat processors wash their beef with ammonia to kill off potentially dangerous bacteria I have had a question looming in my mind. How does ammonia affect the nutrients in the meat? And it's not just beef that is subjected to this chemical cleansing. Chickens are also washed in bleach for similar reasons.

Let's put aside the fact that both substances are considered poisonous. Just consider what that might do to the minerals and vitamins in the meat. Does it alter them? I have a difficult time believing that it doesn't since, I know how easily water-soluble vitamins are destroyed. Has anyone studied it? Does anyone know? And if so, why aren't speaking about it? The fact is that we, the consumers, do not know.

Wouldn't it be easier just to avoid the whole thing? Wouldn't it be easier to not have to worry or wonder, but instead just eat food in its natural state, grown by people who love to grow food in sustainable ways... people who love the animals they are raising so they treat them humanely?

Some time ago, Jane came to see me suffering with severe allergies. We talked about what she was eating and how diet plays a crucial role in building a healthy, balanced immune system. Although she understood what I was saying, she became very upset.

"Look, I get it!" Jane said as she shook her head and curled her shoulders. "But I'm ridiculously busy. I don't have time to change my whole food thing. Honestly, I eat well. Really. It's not that bad that it's making me sick. I'm sure of that."

"Okay," I said. "We'll just do what we can then."

If there's one thing I've learned over the years, it's that you can't force people to be healthy if they don't want to. They may even want to, but for whatever reason, they aren't ready to make that one extra step into taking full responsibility for their well-being. It can be hard to change what you've been doing for years. I also know that for some people, change comes more slowly than for others.

Knowing Jane was desperate, we continued our work together. Many of her symptoms improved, but her allergies just would not let up. Every time she came in not feeling well and she tested positive for some food additive or chemical affecting her, I would gently mention the food subject again.

And once again, I would hear the reasons she could not possibly do what I was suggesting. Until one day, she came in, sat down, and started to cry.

"I don't know what is wrong with me," she said through her tears. "I am so frustrated. I just can't take this anymore. I'm doing everything you say and it's just not getting better."

Here was the moment I had been waiting for. I pointed out there was one change I had recommended to her she had yet to implement.

She took a deep breath, looked at me squarely, and said, "I know. The food."

In that moment, I knew she was ready. I suggested we implement The 21-Day Diet Detox so she could see the effect of eating a diet of food instead of a diet of C.R.A.P. would have on her health. She took a deep breath and agreed reluctantly.

After a few bumpy days, she committed completely to the guidelines of the food program. The first few days she didn't feel well, emailing me frequently, saying how bad she felt, how it wasn't working, etc. I encouraged her to stick with it. I reminded her that thousands of people had done this before and I knew she could too. When she came in at the end of the 21 days, she had a big smile on her face.

"I feel amazing!" she said. "I can't believe the difference it made." She went on to tell me how in just 21 days all of her remaining symptoms improved. We both laughed.

As she walked out the door, she looked over her shoulder and said, "I love/hate when you are right," with a huge smile on her face.

She could no longer deny that what she ate mattered when it came to her health and her body thanked her for making the changes.

Food Intolerance – What Is It and Why Do I Care?

Food intolerances can be a major source of internal stress on the body. Not everyone has a food intolerance affecting his or her health, but if you do, it is essential to identify it and eliminate the offending food from your diet.

A food intolerance occurs when the body reacts to a particular food by waging an immune response that causes inflammation in your system, and that can contribute to almost any health issue.

Many people mistake food intolerances for allergies, thinking it is a pollen that is making their nose run all the time, or they grow accustomed to the symptoms and ignore them. Many, many times when I ask people if they have any foods that are a problem they will identify something, and then when I ask if they eat it, they say yes.

For some people, just one food causes a problem, often a food they eat a lot of. I had a woman come into my practice who tested for sensitivity to dairy. When I told her, her jaw dropped, "How can that be?" she asked. "I grew up on a dairy farm. I have been eating dairy my whole life?"

"Exactly," I explained. Often, the foods we eat the most are what we develop a sensitivity to.

Food intolerances develop when your body creates antibodies to a food, like it would to a virus, such as chickenpox. Antibodies act as the alert system that tells your body there has been a foreign invasion and the immune system must be activated. The problem is that what the immune system is preparing to battle is something that is "supposed" to be good for you.

Although you can become intolerant to anything, the most common foods people react to are foods consumed on a regular basis; wheat, soy, dairy, eggs, nuts, and other grains such as corn.

Although there is not a definitive consensus on the cause of all cases of food intolerance, there are several theories. One such theory, that is supported by what I find in my clinic, is that what we eat has been so vastly altered from its original form, the body no longer recognizes it as food.

When food is combined with chemicals in the form of pesticides, colorings, flavorings, preservatives, heavy metals and other toxins, the body recognizes these foreign substances as a problem, and, in its goal to protect us, creates antibodies to not only the substance, but also the food to which it is attached.

This theory has been supported by recent research pointing to glyphosate as a potential factor in the development of food intolerances.[11]

It is suspected that glyphosates are playing a role in the development of leaky gut. A leaky gut develops when the natural barrier found in a healthy intestine that does not allow food particles that are too large to pass through the intestinal wall and into the bloodstream, is compromised, allowing those larger food particles in. Once the larger particles are in the bloodstream, the body recognizes them as a foreign invader and antibodies are made against the food. Once antibodies are present in high enough numbers an intolerance then develops.

When I have a client who has several food intolerances and becomes reactive to things they eat frequently, my first suspicion is leaky gut.

This was one of the problems I dealt with in my health crisis. I was told I had irritable bowel and would just have to live with it. After living with it for many years, I developed a leaky gut. As a result, I became intolerant to almost every food I was eating: wheat and gluten, oats, corn, dairy, eggs, and soy. Leaky gut is very slow to heal and the dietary requirements for healing have a tremendous effect on a person's quality of life. This makes paying attention to digestive upset before leaky gut develops a much better strategy than trying to control it once it surfaces.

Any time there is prolonged inflammation in the intestines, there is a risk of developing leaky gut. Inflammation in the intestines can be from many sources. Sometimes a food intolerance can actually be the cause of the development of leaky gut. However, chronic intestinal infections that are undiagnosed and untreated, a buildup of chemicals or heavy metals in the body and chronic improper pH in the stomach can all lead to inflammation and a subsequent breakdown of the barrier if left unaddressed.

A food intolerance can be a primary factor in your health issues, or it can be one of many contributing factors. When it is one of many factors, it can be even trickier to identify on your own, as eliminating the food itself will not "solve" the problem.

I had a client come in complaining of acid reflux and severe allergies that she was treating with medication. Testing her, we found a pathogenic bug in her intestines, and two food intolerances: gluten and chocolate. This was when I took a deep breath and paused.

"Well I have some good news. I am pretty sure I can help you, but also some not so good news. You are going to have to stop eating gluten and chocolate." I was shocked to find that chocolate was a problem, as it has rarely shown up as one.

As we worked to eliminate the bug in her intestines, she worked to remove the gluten and chocolate from her diet. Eliminating gluten was pretty easy for her. The chocolate, however, took a bit longer. Even though her symptoms improved after eliminating the bug and gluten, it wasn't until she was able to stay off chocolate for several weeks that her stomach pain completely resolved. And not only did her stomach pain resolve but she also no longer takes any medications, not even her daily allergy pill.

If a food intolerance is a primary factor in your health challenge, then removing the offending food from your diet will resolve your issues. However, as with the young woman mentioned above, more often than not, there are several contributing factors and eliminating a problem food alone will not completely resolve the issue. In her case, we had to first eliminate her immune challenge, the fungal overgrowth as well as get the gluten and chocolate out of her diet.

It takes about three months for the antibodies to a food to disappear from your system. That's why it is so important to be vigilant about eliminating the offending food. In some cases, the food in question can be successfully reintroduced back into the diet as long as it is in its natural form. For others, food intolerances are more permanent. If you know you have a food intolerance, such as dairy, take a break from it 100 percent for three months. Then, add in some raw unpasteurized dairy and see if you get a reaction. If you don't, you may be able to add it back in its raw form in small amounts. If you do react, that is a food you should avoid at all costs.

When you do reintroduce a food, pay close attention. Symptoms of food intolerance vary and can contribute to almost any health problem. Some of the most common are; itchiness on the body, rashes or acne breakouts, bloating, or other digestive problems including irritable bowel syndrome, headaches, and increased pain anywhere in the body, even autoimmune diseases. A reaction might also present like a cold, with congestion, and aching. In some people, a shift in mood can be a sign. Any new symptom or recurring aggravation that occurs within three days of reintroducing a questionable food should be suspect.

Eating organic foods not exposed to pesticides, and foods in their natural form, free of processing, can do a lot to protect you and your gut health. Once you have cleaned out your system, as you will do with the The 21-Day Diet Detox, you will more readily notice if a food that you add back in your diet causes a reaction. When you eat something on a regular basis that is an irritant, your overall homeostasis will adapt to the chronic stress the food places on your system and you won't fully notice its effect. Once you abstain for a minimum of 21 days, you'll be able to truly assess how much of a problem a specific food is for your body. Eliminate problem foods from your diet and you will make huge strides toward feeling better.

Pay attention to your body! Don't ignore even those tolerable symptoms you experience when you eat a particular food. You may be creating inflammation in your body that is contributing to your not feeling well or, even worse, the development of disease.

Gluten Sensitivities: Real Thing or the Latest Food Fad?

Gluten (from Latin *gluten*, "glue") is a protein found in the grains wheat, rye, barley, spelt, kamut, and oats, often as a result of cross contamination. Its role in the life cycle of plants is to power the sprouting process. Gluten gives elasticity to dough, helping it to rise and keep its shape. Hence, the reason gluten-containing breads are soft and chewy as opposed to their gluten-free cardboard-like counterparts.

Gluten has always been in grains. It is a natural substance that makes it possible for the plant to germinate. Grains, particularly wheat, have been a major part of our diet, in some parts of the world, since the dawn of civilization.

If humans have been eating gluten-containing grains for thousands of years, how is it that it's become such a problem? Has it really become a problem, or is this just the latest craze of ever-evolving food fads?

Unfortunately, it is not a fad. Gluten intolerance, also known as gluten sensitivity is a very real problem. As a matter of fact, the number of gluten sensitive people is rising so fast one might call it an epidemic. The reasons for this "epidemic" are complex and varied. Let's start with what gluten intolerance is and why it matters to you and your health, if you have it.

First of all, understand that many health professionals do not recognize gluten intolerance as an actual thing. However, they do recognize an extreme gluten reaction that causes an autoimmune disorder known as celiac disease. Celiac disease is a genetic disorder that results in damage to the lining of the small intestine when exposed to gluten.

According to the Mayo clinic website, "Celiac disease is on the rise." Mayo Clinic research suggests the disease is becoming a major public health issue. Although the cause is unknown, "celiac disease is four times more common now than 60 years ago, and affects about one in 100 people."[12]

Gluten intolerance is different from celiac disease. And, regardless of the fact that many medical doctors believe celiac disease is the only real form of gluten intolerance, research and clinical experience confirm that other forms are a real problem and can have very serious health consequences.

Gluten intolerance is defined as having an "immune response to gluten." It is different from what is called an allergy due to the fact that different immune cells are reacting.

Often, with gluten intolerance, a person will experience inflammation that affects some tissue in the body. This is why gluten can affect more than just the digestive tract as it does in celiac disease. In fact, much of the recent research on gluten intolerance is correlating the affects of gluten on neurological tissue and the role it may play in autoimmune diseases.[13, 14]

Research has found gluten intolerance may also play a role in the development of many neurological disorders, such as multiple sclerosis (MS), Parkinson's Disease, Lou Gehrig's disease, and many other auto-immune diseases beyond just celiac, including but not limited to Hashimoto's Thyroiditis.

A few months ago, I had a young girl come into my clinic who was suffering with severe migraines. In fact, she'd had so many the previous month, she had taken 22 capsules of iMatrex, a strong medication used to help migraine sufferers.

When she mentioned to her doctor that she'd taken that many in one month, he was extremely upset because iMatrex taken that often can have serious negative health effects, particularly for her liver. But without it, the migraines threatened to take over her life. She was losing her ability to plan or imagine a future because she never knew when a debilitating headache would hit.

When I tested her, I found gluten was a problem. She cut gluten out of her diet and her headaches drastically decreased. From 22 capsules in one month to two. I don't know about you, but I call that a miracle! This was further confirmed when she was accidentally exposed to gluten, as can happen, and the frequent migraines returned. The correlation was irrefutable.

I have seen gluten sensitivity play a role in everything from skin rashes to hormonal imbalances, autoimmune diseases, arthritis and other chronic inflammatory diseases, brain degenerative diseases, back pain, digestive problems, chronic fatigue, depression, and anxiety just to mention a few.

Often, we don't even know what health issue is being aggravated until gluten is removed from the diet. When removed 100 percent for a minimum of three weeks, we are able to see what symptoms disappear, or re-appear once the gluten is reintroduced.

Clearly, not every disease progression has gluten intolerance as part of its development, but I am willing to say that if gluten intolerance is one of your underlying issues, you will not heal until you get it completely out of your diet.

While gluten has always been in grain and humans have been exposed to it as long as we have been eating grains, several things have changed that are fueling the current rise in the number of people experiencing intolerance:

- The way we harvest our grain is not the same as it was in years past. Classically, grains were harvested in a way that allowed sprouting to occur as a natural part of the process. In modern agriculture, the germ is removed while harvesting, which halts sprouting. Gluten is the protein in grains that promotes sprouting, and when sprouting is halted, the protein is not utilized. Because the protein has not been used, the amount of gluten in the grain is higher than it traditionally had been, exposing the consumer to a higher level of gluten.
- Over the years, a greater amount of gluten has been bred into wheat, leading to the development of higher-gluten flour. Wheat has been hybridized so much that it is fundamentally a different substance from *original* wheat.
- The way we make dough has also been affected. It used to be that, in the making of dough, grains were sprouted prior to making them into flour, and flour was fermented prior to baking. Both sprouting and fermentation decrease the level of gluten in the final bread product. These traditional bread-making steps have been eliminated, resulting in higher gluten levels in our flour-containing food products.
- To top it off, a food additive called deamidated gliadin is being added to food, in some of the most unexpected places such as in commercially raised turkeys with added flavors. It is proving to be a very high irritant to the human body; unfortunately, once a reaction to deamidated gliadin has developed, a cross reaction to gluten is likely.

If you suffer from back pain, arthritis, fibromyalgia, heart burn, irritable bowel and chronic digestive upset, brain fog, depression, or anxiety disorders, A.D.D. and other learning disabilities, any auto immune disorder especially Hashimoto's thyroiditis, disorders such as early Alzheimer's, Lou Gehrig's disease, multiple sclerosis, or any other degenerative brain disease, you may have a gluten intolerance that is contributing to your health issue.

One area of concern I cannot stress enough is the connection between gluten intolerance and moods. I rarely find a female who has been experiencing depression and anxiety for many years who does not have a gluten sensitivity.

I had a woman who came to my office off and on for a few years and I noticed that our talks often turned to her moods. She would talk about her bouts of depression, anger, and anxiety.

During the time we were working together, I took part in a seminar on gluten intolerance and learned that gluten often caused emotional upset. Shortly after that seminar, she came to see me again.

"Oh God, Cari," she squeaked out, tears threatening to spill from her eyes. "I am out of control. I don't know what is going on with me!"

Knowing she'd been in counseling for 20 years, give or take, I was taken aback by her emotional volatility.

"Tell me what's happening," I said, moving in to comfort her.

"I think I'm going crazy! I was so insane yesterday; I actually threw my cell phone across the room and broke it."

"What happened to upset you so much?" I asked.

"Nothing. Really. Nothing. That's the thing that has me so freaked out!"

She suddenly went very quiet and I knew there was more to come.

"There's this thing. This thing that happened when I was a kid and I…I can't seem to get a handle on it. Now my husband is threatening to leave if I don't get on medication. Even my therapist thinks I should be taking meds. But I just don't want to go down that road. I just don't want to."

It was a plaintive cry for help and knowing she had been on anxiety medication before, and that it had negative side effects for her, I understood her desire to avoid them. My heart was breaking for her.

Remembering what I had just learned about gluten and moods, and that she had tested sensitive to gluten but had yet to take it out of her diet 100 percent, I decided to bring it up again.

"Listen," I said. "I think it might be helpful for you to get off gluten. Remember, we talked about it before and I just learned how much it can affect your mood. Why don't you go off of it completely and let's see if we can get to the bottom of your emotional upset."

As is often the case when someone gets to this point, she was willing to try anything. So she exorcised gluten from her diet 100 percent. About three months later, she came into my office wearing a huge smile.

"Wow!" I said, jokingly shielding my eyes from the glow of her aura,"What's up?"

"I retired my therapist. His services are no longer needed!"

Since ridding her diet of gluten, the unresolved emotional issues ceased bothering her. Her moods became stable and her husband stopped insisting she take medication. Her anger had subsided and she felt balanced and calm again. Now, all the years of work she had done with her therapist could take effect.

I often see stories like this in my practice. I have also experienced the effects of gluten on brain function up close and personal. As a matter of fact, my entire paternal family on my fathers side and I are gluten intolerant.

I was the first to kick off the diagnosis party, followed eventually by each family member being tested as a result of some health challenge. And though we all tested positive, the symptoms for each of us were different. My symptoms, when exposed, are much more brain-related—severe brain fog and memory loss are the primary symptoms I experience that tell me I have been exposed.

Because gluten intolerance has become such a broad-reaching problem, I recommend most people decrease their exposure. This will protect you and your children from developing an intolerance in the future.

Following The 21-Day Diet Detox is a great first step to detecting if gluten is a problem for you. After being off gluten for the 21 days, you will be able to see if it is affecting you when you add it back in. Confirming if you have a gluten intolerance can be done with a blood test as well. However, not just any blood test will do. The standard of medical care in America at this time is to test for antibodies to one, maybe two parts of a gluten molecule, which often results in false negative tests.

The most comprehensive test done by a lab in southern California called CYREX Labs, tests for reactions to several more parts of the gluten molecule, so it has a higher likelihood of identifying a problem if it exists. The test costs $325 at this writing and is worth every penny if you are having a health challenge that gluten could be aggravating or even causing.

Avoiding gluten can be tricky at first. But once you educate yourself about the hidden sources and you feel the benefits of a gluten-free diet, the practice will become second nature.

Avoiding gluten is a commitment. It takes time to educate yourself about how to be truly 100 percent gluten free. As we mentioned earlier, gluten is hidden in some pretty unexpected places, such as your skin and hair care products. Education about how to be gluten free is beyond the scope of this book. However, the good news is that there are many resources on the Internet and many books written on the subject. So the information and support is readily available and abundant.

Remember, there is no such thing as being *mostly* gluten-free. It is an all-in affair. Even one molecule of gluten can activate an immune response, and that response can last in your body for several months. The consequences to your health trump the short-term gratification. Skip the cookie and live a long, vibrant life!

END NOTES

1. Business Dictionary, s.v. "food," accessed August 23, 2015, http://www.businessdictionary.com/definition/food.html#ixzz3hOa8x3QN
2. "Statistics FAQs," accessed September 1, 2015, https://www.tfi.org/statistics/statistics-faqs
3. Stephanie Strom, "Misgivings About How a Weed Killer Affects the Soil," The New York Times, September 19, 2013, accessed August 23, 2015, http://www.nytimes.com/2013/09/20/business/misgivings-about-how-a-weed-killer-affects-the-soil.html?_r=1
4. Brian Halweil, "Still No Free Lunch: Nutrient Levels in U.S. Food Supply Eroded by Pursuit of High Yields," The Organic Center, September, 2007, accessed August 23, 2015, https://www.organic-center.org/reportfiles/Yields2Pager.pdf
5. Michael Alavanja, "Pesticides Use and Exposure Extensive Worldwide," *Reviews on Environmental Health* 24, no. 4 (October-December 2009): 303, accessed August 23, 2015, http://www.ncbi.nlm.nih.gov/pmc/articles/PMC2946087/

6. "Human Health Issues," last modified October 17, 2014, accessed August 23, 2015, http://www.epa.gov/pesticides/health/human.htm

7. Karen Feldscher, "Toxic Chemicals Linked to Brain Disorders in Children," *Harvard Gazette* (February 14, 2014): 1, accessed August 23, 2015, http://news.harvard.edu/gazette/story/2014/02/toxic-chemicals-linked-to-brain-disorders-in-children/

8. "Who We Are: Annual Letter 2012," accessed August 23, 2015, http://www.gatesfoundation.org/who-we-are/resources-and-media/annual-letters-list/annual-letter-2012

9. Jason Kane, "Health Costs: How the U.S. Compares With Other Countries," PBS.org, October 22, 2012, accessed August 23, 2015, http://www.pbs.org/newshour/rundown/health-costs-how-the-us-compares-with-other-countries/

10. Ryan Jaslow, "U.S. Health 'mediocre' Compared to Other Wealthy Countries," CBS News.com, July 10, 2013, accessed August 23, 2015, http://www.cbsnews.com/news/us-health-mediocre-compared-to-other-wealthy-countries/

11. Anthony Samsel and Stephanie Seneff, "Glyphosate's Suppression of Cytochrome P450 Enzymes and Amino Acid Biosynthesis by the Gut Microbiome: Pathways to Modern Diseases," Entropy 2013 15, no. 1099-4300 (April, 2013): 1416-1463, accessed August 23, 2015, https://groups.csail.mit.edu/sls/publications/2013/Seneff_Entropy-15-01416.pdf

12. "Celiac Disease: On the Rise," *Discovery's Edge,* July 2010, accessed August 27, 2015, http://www.mayo.edu/research/discoverys-edge/celiac-disease-rise

13. Kate Solomon, "Do You Have Gluten Sensitivity or an Autoimmune Disease?" Huffington Post, October 30,2014, Updated December 30, 2014, accessed August 27, 2015, http://www.huffing tonpost.com/kate-solomon/do-you-have-gluten-sensit_b_6021306.html

14. Jessica R. Jackson, William W. Eaton, Nicola G. Cascella, Alessio Fasano, and Deanna L. Kelly, "Neurologic and Psychiatric Manifestations of Celiac Disease and Gluten Sensitivity," Psychiatric Quarterly 83, no. 1 (March, 2012): 91-102, accessed August 27, 2015, http://www.ncbi.nlm.nih.gov/pmc/articles/PMC3641836/

CHAPTER 5

Who's Minding the Store: Enrichment, Additives, and Oversight

The Enrichment and Fortification of Food

Vitamin:
- any group of organic compounds that are essential for normal growth and nutrition and are required in small quantities in the diet because they cannot be synthesized by the body.[1]

Minerals:
- any of the inorganic elements, as calcium, iron, magnesium, potassium, or sodium, that are essential to the functioning of the human body and are obtained from foods.

Vitamins and minerals were "discovered" as man altered or restricted food and then began to get sick. This phenomenon made scientists of the time curious as to the cause.

The case of vitamin C is a perfect example. In the 1550s, Jacques Cartier, an established explorer, noted that the sailors under his command who had consumed oranges, limes, and berries did not get scurvy, and those who already had the disease and were ingesting these fruits had a much higher rate of recovery.

But it wasn't until 1742 that it was determined there was a definite connection between the diet and scurvy. Lemon juice was given to people who suffered with scurvy for several doses and they healed!

While this method of treatment became common at sea, its applicable dietary benefits did not translate to the rest of the population. In the late 1800s, infants were dying from scurvy at record rates and no one could determine why. It wasn't determined until the early 1900s when studies showed that vitamin C, naturally found in babies' milk was being destroyed in the routine pasteurization process.

Today, the food we eat is more often than not altered from its original form and, as I have stated, this processing of food has led to a decline in the nutrient content of what we are eating. Food enrichment and fortification is food manufacturers' and our government's attempt at countering the negative affect of this. But like the chemicals in commercial fertilizer, what they are adding is only a Band-Aid to the problem, not a solution.

Enrichment is the process of adding back nutrients, naturally found in a food, that were destroyed in processing. Pasteurized milk is a good example of an enriched product. During the pasteurization process, vitamin D and A are destroyed so they are added back into the pasteurized milk prior to selling. Ironically, the final enriched product has less nutrition than its natural counterpart had.

Fortification is the practice of adding nutrients to food products that are not found in the food in its original state. Orange juice that has vitamin D added to it is a good example of fortification, as vitamin D is not naturally found in oranges.

Adding nutrients to food that are not naturally found in the food, is a perfect example of how we have lost the understanding that nutrients act in synergy rather than in isolated form. In order to function, the body uses a complex of nutrients. Bones are not made from calcium alone. To make bone, calcium, magnesium and vitamin D, protein, fats, trace minerals, and other co-factors are also needed.

The practice of altering food by adding in nutrients began when the processing of food first became broad reaching in this country. In the late 1800s, when a new type of flour mill was introduced, called roller mills, the bran and germ began to be removed almost entirely from wheat flour. Unfortunately, the bran and germ of wheat contain the bulk of the nutrition. With the loss of these parts of the grain, B vitamins, fiber, fat-soluble vitamins, and essential amino acids are lost, leaving only the starch and sugars.

The first head of the Food and Drug Administration (FDA), Dr. Harvey Wiley, who advocated for pure foods and drugs in the United States, tried to outlaw refined, bleached white flour because of the loss of nutrition that resulted while making it. He lost the battle, however, and was replaced as head of the FDA in 1912.

When the United States exported these new milling systems into Great Britain, there was backlash from the British Medical Society over concerns that the roller mills produced less nutritious flour.[2]

In the late 1930s, there was concern raised about the nutritional health of Americans when it was found that the overall health of the young men enlisting for service during World War II was poor. In 1938, the AMA Council of Foods and Nutrition endorsed the addition of nutrients to foods to counter this problem. By the end of 1942, 75% of white bread was fortified with thiamin, niacin, iron, and riboflavin that were made in a lab, and the accepted broad-reaching enrichment of food began.

In the case of minerals, the minerals added in to fortify and enrich food are often in the form found in rocks, instead of food.

For instance, calcium carbonate, the form of calcium found in cement, is used to fortify food products, and is also used in many dietary supplements. There is recent evidence that the plaque found in our arteries in heart disease and our brains in some neurological diseases may be due to the consumption of nonabsorbable forms of minerals that are added to what we eat, especially minerals like iron and calcium carbonate.

When enriching first began, it seemed to work. The incidence of the diseases that were increasing due to the processing of flour and the pasteurizing of milk did decrease. However, when we look at the overall health of our citizens today, obviously it did not really solve the problem. If the enrichment and fortification process was adding in all that was being lost during processing, then we would not be continuing to discover "new" nutrients that are needed for our health.

The fact is, none of the "new" discoveries about food and nutrition are new. The human body has the same needs now as it did thousands of years ago. All that the human body needs to stay healthy can be found in pure food, air, and water, in their original whole form. This has to be true because, long before food altering existed, these bodies evolved using food to thrive—real food, not the enriched or fortified versions we are being sold today. When foodstuff is enriched, what is added in is only a portion of what was lost. What is added in is an inferior grade known as an isolate form of vitamin and/or a rock form of mineral.

Can't I Just Take a Vitamin Pill and Call It a Day?

Dr. Royal Lee warned that just as the chemist cannot create life, neither can he create a complex vitamin, the life element in foods and nutrition. This is a mystery the chemist has not solved and probably never will, and the synthetic vitamins he creates on the basis of chemical formulas bear as much resemblance to the real thing as a robot does to a living man, lacking an elusive quality that chemistry cannot supply.[3]

It is true that sometimes, especially when we are under extreme stress, or when our body is healing, taking a vitamin and mineral supplement is necessary and can be a really good idea. However, taking a vitamin to counter-act a nutrient-poor, chemical-rich diet, is not a sound strategy. The vitamin and minerals may help your body counter the negative affects of the choices you are making, but it can never fully replace the benefit of a life supported by healthy nutritious food.

If taking a supplement feels like a good idea, then there is something really important for you to understand. NOT ALL VITAMIN SUPPLEMENTS ARE THE SAME, and when it comes to your health and well-being, it makes a big difference what kind of supplement you choose.

In the world of nutrition, there are two basic categories of vitamin and mineral supplements: 1) those that are created in a lab and are referred to as isolates, or nutraceuticals, and 2) those made by concentrating food, known as whole food supplements.

A nutraceutical is a blend of the words nutrition and pharmaceutical. It is a nutritional supplement that has been manufactured in a lab. Vitamins, when found in nature, are in a complex structure of other things besides just what we call the vitamin itself. When we take a vitamin that has been made in a lab, we are ingesting only part of the complex of how that nutrient naturally occurs in the food we eat. What has been observed in the human body is that when we take nutrients in isolation of their co-factors, you are putting yourself at risk for creating a new and different kind of imbalance in the body or, in other words, a new health problem.

Let me put this in terms that may be simpler to understand. You decide to bake a cake for a bake sale your daughter is having at school. You go to the store to buy what you need and they are having a great sale on sugar, so you decide to get a whole lot of it. You are so excited to have so much sugar you start to bake like crazy. After a while, you notice you are starting to run low on eggs, you have so much sugar and you are baking for a good cause, so you continue baking, but without the eggs. Now you are still making a dessert, but it is a little more like fudge than a cake. This continues and eventually, you run out of more and more ingredients, but you still have an abundance of sugar; so now, all you can make is caramelized sugar candy.

This is what it is like in the body when you take an isolate form of a vitamin. You may get those B vitamins you need; however, you are not getting all the other co-factors necessary to fully support your system. Eventually, you run the risk of running out of one or more of those co-factors and ending up with a new kind of health challenge—one that may be more difficult to treat because no one has "discovered" the thing you are lacking.

Taking isolates predisposes you to two potential problems: one, creating a deficiency of another nutrient, and two, not actually giving your body what it needs to correct its health problem. If, when you brush your teeth and your toothbrush turns pink from bleeding gums, you may have a low-level vitamin C deficiency or scurvy affecting your health. I bet if you look at that super everything vitamin pill you take every day, ascorbic acid, the non-food form of vitamin C, is on the list of ingredients in high amounts.

It is often confusing when we consider whether or not we should take supplements because one day there is a study touting their benefits and the next, you'll read about how they increase your chance of developing a disease.

One such article found in the *New York Times* titled, "Don't Take Your Supplements," by Paula Offit, published: June 8, 2013, quotes study after study citing the increased risk of death from taking certain supplements.[4]

Another review, published in 2005 in the *Annals of Internal Medicine*, found that in 19 trials of nearly 136,000 people, supplemental vitamin E increased mortality. These studies are enough to put you off that vitamin pill for months. However, it is isolates that are being studied not whole food supplements.[5]

When you decide to take a vitamin or mineral supplement, make sure you are taking one that is made from food. You aren't going to get sick from taking a pill of concentrated beets and carrots.

Additives: The C.R.A.P. of It All.

In one way or another, everything about the food we eat has dramatically shifted in the last 100 years. Everything from the way it is grown, harvested, processed, sold, packaged, stored, or cooked has changed. But the greatest, most disturbing change to date is the advent of the chemical food additive, chemicals that are legally allowed to be added to our food during processing.

As of this writing, August 2015, there are over 14,000 chemicals that are approved additives, 3000 of which you will never see on the label, because food regulations do not require that they be listed. These 3000 chemicals are on the government's so-called GRAS list, Generally Recognized as Safe.

When food is altered, processed in some way, and chemicals are added, nutrients are denatured and destroyed. With the addition of chemicals to our food source, our body now has the added burden of having to bio-transform and eliminate the chemicals, all of which require nutrients.

When I first learned about the GRAS list, I assumed that when I saw artificial ingredients on a list of ingredients, it meant there were one or two things added in. I had no idea the magnitude of what that little phrase could mean. Then I read Eric Schlosser's book, *Fast Food Nation*. In his book, he lists the ingredients in a Burger King milkshake that will never appear on the label. It was staggering information.

There are over 40 chemicals, with names like amyl acetate, or benzyl isobutyrate. There is even some solvent, just in case you need to clean a paintbrush while enjoying your BK shake!

But Burger King isn't alone here, and it isn't my intention to single them out. This is an industry standard that crosses the field from fast food to processed *health foods. Processed health foods?* That's an oxymoron if ever I heard one! If you don't believe me, start reading the labels.

I had several clients who were really into one of the latest frozen yogurt companies. They loved to take their kids there after school for a fun family outing. *Frozen yogurt – what could be wrong with that, right? Isn't it a health food?* In testing their children, I found that chemicals were part of their health issues. Investigating the source, just out of curiosity, I looked up the yogurt ingredients. What I found was there wasn't much *frozen yogurt* in the product, mostly just chemicals: some non-organic, non-fat pasteurized dairy, and a whole lot of chemicals.

So, I started to wonder, "If the GRAS chemicals are generally recognized as safe, what are the other thousands of chemicals added to our food considered? GRAD? Generally Recognized as Dangerous?"

I also wondered, "What determines whether a particular chemical makes the cut for the GRAS list and is put in our food unlabeled?"

So, I did a little research, which, by the way, is pretty easy to do. Just go to the FDA's website, and you'll find it all there in plain English.

According to the FDA, chemicals on the GRAS list are chemicals that are generally and widely considered safe, or have been added to food prior to 1958. No research needed, they just had to have been around for a long time or have to be "regarded as safe." Who determines that is up for discussion.

In 1998, when it was discovered that a chemical on the GRAS list was actually dangerous, the list was updated and reviewed. That gave me a little peace, but not much. Because, truthfully, the chemical identified on the list had been in use, remember, since before 1958, and it wasn't until the '90s that it was identified as a problem. That's scary. Also, I could find no research that looked at the safety of combining these chemicals together. So how do they know that all 40 of those chemicals in the BK shake are actually safe when consumed together?

For a long time, cigarettes were considered safe, even touted by doctors as a health and weight loss aid in magazine ads. Hydrogenated oils (trans-fats) the main ingredient in Crisco and margarine, were introduced in 1911. It wasn't until the 1990s that it became required to list trans-fats on the label in a separate category, even though they have been known since the 50s to contribute to the development of heart disease and elevated cholesterol among a host of other potentially serious health problems. So much for the rule, *if it's been used a long time, and by large numbers of people it must be safe.*

Today, products containing hydrogenated oils (trans-fats) are still allowed in food but must be singled out on the label, unless, of course, there is less than 1% added; then, manufacturers are allowed to tout that the food "contains no trans-fats." It must be a math thing!

So what about the other 11,000 G.R.A.D. chemicals, as I call them, added to our food? How is it determined what and how much of a chemical is safe to put in our food. It is decided based on "probable consumer intake." The FDA and US Department of Human Services protects us from too much of a "bad thing" by estimating how much you are likely to eat, compared "to the level at which adverse effects are observed in toxicological studies." Simply stated on the FDA website, "the dose makes the poison."

Hold on a minute! How do they *estimate* how much of any substance one person will eat? I know I'm not eating my chemical allotment, so statistically does that mean if I'm not eating my share that someone else is? How can you determine what amount is safe for a child of four versus a 250-pound man?

In my opinion, the logic behind "the dose makes the poison" is flawed. How can the consumer know if they are getting too high a dose? The example the FDA uses in their argument is that even too much water can cause you to get sick. Got it...too much of anything can be harmful for your health. I agree.

But I am aware and can control how much water I consume. There is no way for me to know what or how much of these chemicals I am ingesting. My only control is to stop eating foods that contain them, altogether.

We are being exposed to chemicals at record levels. These chemicals do NOTHING good for you. They do not promote your health, they do not promote better function of your organs, and they do not make you thin. They do, however, replace important nutrients in your food and add extra work for your body by increasing the effort your liver and other organs need to exert to keep your body running efficiently. And, in fact, many researchers are blaming them as the cause of numerous diseases as well as possibly playing a role in the rising obesity epidemic. I know I see a correlation between chemicals and weight issues all the time in my clinic.

So, why eat them? Why not choose to avoid them altogether?

If we choose to keep eating processed food laced with chemicals, then the best we can do is hope that we will not develop some disease that we find out was associated with some chemical we were exposed to.

Chemicals are everywhere in our environment, and we cannot immediately control what we are exposed to out in the world. It is impossible. But we can control what we eat. We can do our best to make sure we are eating nutritious food that is low in chemicals; eliminating one more thing with which our bodies must contend. When we do that, we are better equipped to support our bodies in dealing with the chemicals we may be exposed to that are out of our immediate control.

Regulation, Big Business, & Your Food: Who's Watching Out for You?

Government agencies, such as the Food and Drug Administration (FDA) and the Environmental Protection Agency (EPA), were created to make sure the food, water, and drugs we consume are safe. The problem arises around what the definition of safe is and how much influence food manufacturers have over our government agencies.

Let's use fluoride as an example. There is a type of fluoride, Sulfuryl Fluoride, which was developed as a fumigant, a substance used to eradicate pests, in the 1950s. This form of fluoride was banned for use in food by the EPA "Under no circumstances should Vikane™ (the name sulfuryl fluoride was trademarked as) be used on raw agricultural food commodities, foods, feeds, or medicinal products destined for human or animal."[6]

This decision was based on the levels of fluoride remaining in the food after using the fumigant being above approved safe levels.

Then in 2004, the EPA did a complete about-face and approved the same product released under a different name to be used in 40 postharvest products. They did this by raising the levels of fluoride that they recommend as safe for human consumption. By 2005, the EPA went on to approve its use in more than 900 products, again raising the "safe exposure levels" in some cases to ten times higher levels. In many cases, these levels were scientifically proven to be toxic.[7]

Today, the EPA is reconsidering its position. According to the EPA's website, "The U.S. Environmental Protection Agency has re-evaluated the current science on fluoride and is taking steps to begin a phased-down withdrawal of the pesticide sulfuryl fluoride"[8]

Why the back and forth? The producer of Vikane spent years convincing the EPA to approve Vikane's use in food. Then, as stated on the EPA own website "In 2004, the Fluoride Action Network (FAN) filed an objection to the sulfuryl fluoride tolerances and requested a hearing. FAN's objections rest on their belief that fluoride exposure is not safe under the FFDCA. EPA's Office of Pesticide Programs (OPP) has updated its assessment of the risks of sulfuryl fluoride as part of its response to the FAN objections"[9]

Did anyone notice the dates? In 2004, FAN brought its lawsuit. In 2005, the EPA increased its approval for use in food. It is now 2015, and on their own website, the EPA states that the objections raised by FAN are affecting their decision to revise their recommendations. That is 11 years later. That is 11 years of toxic exposure due to bureaucratic delays.

A similar thing is happening with the fluoride added to our drinking water. There is much controversy as to whether adding fluoride to our drinking water is a good idea from a health perspective. However, if we leave that debate aside, and just look at the type of fluoride being added to our water, you will get a better understanding of why we cannot rely on our political system to protect us.

Labeling Laws Can Be Deceiving

The labeling laws in this country are not as straightforward as you would expect. In many cases, labeling laws are nonexistent. In some cases, labels are flat-out misleading. This is one of the things that makes it difficult to know how much C.R.A.P. you're eating.

For example, as I mentioned, trans fats can be added to a food in small amounts and the manufacturer is still allowed to say "zero trans fats" on the front label of the product. That's the power of the lobbyist, and it is one of the huge problems in this country when it comes to our food. There's a lot of money at stake in the food manufacturing business, and many manufacturers use whatever power they have to look out for their interests.

Why would some food manufacturers spend millions of dollars fighting against labeling genetically modified foods? What could possibly be wrong with telling the consumer what has been done to the products they buy?

If we prefer *not* to buy food that has been genetically altered, isn't that our right? The state of Vermont recently passed a law requiring the labeling of GMO foods, and as this book is being written in August of 2015, the state is in court fighting a multimillion-dollar lawsuit to defend the law.

Let's examine labels further, starting with "organic." In a great moment in our food history, the U.S. government established the USDA organic labeling law in 1990. The law set a standard that would assure the public that if they chose to consume food labeled "organic," they would be eating something that had been grown using sustainable chemical-free methods. In the 1990s, the organic food industry was a billion dollar industry. Over the past 15 years, it has become a $30 billion industry. As a result, pressure was applied and laws have been modified to allow previously prohibited synthetic substances to be used in foods labeled organic. Did you ever wonder why organic food started showing up in more and more stores, including the mega supermarkets? These changes make it easier for large food growers to comply with the "new" weaker organic standards. And, to make it worse, the latest changes were made behind closed doors without any input from oversight committees.[12] This sets the stage for future changes to the law without any review. The result of all this is that unfortunately, you can't rely on food labeled organic to mean that they are nutritious and chemically free anymore.[13]

Buying organic anything is still better than not buying organic, though. By eating organic, whether the food is grown using the guidelines of the old laws or newer more lenient ones, and whether it is processed or not, you will be exposed to fewer chemicals overall. The same is true for the meat you buy. When you buy organic, the meat will come from animals that have been treated somewhat more humanely.

"Free range" is a wonderful term that suggests animals enjoying a bucolic landscape. But guess what? No law exists regarding the use of this term. The food producers decide what to label free range with one exception. In order for a chicken to qualify for the free-range label, it must be "allowed access to the outside." The USDA does not specify the frequency of access or size of the outside range, nor does it specify the duration of time an animal must have this access.[14]

Grass-Fed has some labeling requirements but they are a little vague. According to the Environmental Working Group (EWG), a consumer watchdog website devoted to informing us about chemicals in our food and skin care, the "USDA's grass-fed marketing standard… does not necessarily mean that the animals spent their entire lives in pastures or on rangeland. Some cattle marketed as USDA grass-fed actually spend part of their lives in confined pens or feedlots." This is an unhealthy, inhumane environment, to say the least.[15]

Last but not least, we find the much-used word *natural* on our labels. Ever wonder exactly what that means? Want to try to figure it out? If so, well… good luck! According to the FDA's own website, they do not even seem to know.

Take a look at this direct quote:

> What is the meaning of "natural" on the label of food?
>
> From a food science perspective, it is difficult to define a food product that is "natural" because the food has probably been processed and is no longer the product of the earth. That said, FDA has not developed a definition for use of the term natural or its derivatives. However, the agency has not objected to the use of the term if the food does not contain added color, artificial flavors, or synthetic substances.[16]

So does that mean organic food is not natural, since we already established organic can contain synthetic chemicals?

The basic truth is that labels are often vague, confusing and contain loopholes, which, I will venture to say, often are found and used. So, you have to be careful. You cannot trust that the words used on labels will mean what they seem to mean.

This information can be depressing and overwhelming but it is important to understand that labels can and often do mislead you, that there are thousands of poorly tested chemicals in your food, and that the government is not able or willing to protect you from them.

It is important info to learn so you are motivated and empowered to make new informed choices to protect your health. This way will require some learning on your part, some changes in habits, both in food choices and where you allocate your funds. However, once made, these changes can and will become an easy and pleasurable part of your life.

The Research …or Lack Thereof

Have you ever wondered why the information out there about nutrition is so confusing? One source says one thing, while another source says another. It can be infuriating. Eat eggs…don't eat eggs.

Fat is bad for you... you need fat for good health. This is the best water to drink, but wait, actually, now this type of water is better.

Everybody has an opinion.

Why is this? Why is there so much confusion about what our bodies need to be healthy? We have been around for thousands of years. Doesn't it seem like we should have it figured out by now? Yes it does, and I believe the answer to why we still have so much confusion goes back to something mentioned earlier. We have forgotten the purpose of food, and, in the process, we have forgotten what food is.

You see, Americans love to take things apart. We love to dissect things to gain a deeper understanding of what they are, which is great. However, we often forget to put them back together. Once taken apart, we start to relate to them as individual pieces instead of parts of a whole.

Nowhere is this more evident than in medicine. There are specialists for every part of the body. We often behave as if each part can function on its own without any connection to the rest. In nutrition, we have done a similar thing. We take food apart, identify what we think is important, and throw the rest out. The problem is you cannot do that. Just as you cannot take the body apart and expect it to function the same way, you cannot take nutrition apart and expect it to have the same effect.

For example, what we call vitamin C is really ascorbic acid. Ascorbic acid is a part of the vitamin C complex. It is the outer shell of the whole nutrient complex and it does not have the same effect in the body as the whole nutrient. This is why ascorbic acid won't cure scurvy but a food like a lime will. The food has the whole complex of nutrients that support the effect vitamin C has in the body.

When you read about nutrition studies, you are not reading about the effects of food on the body, but rather the effect of an isolated part of food on the body. Often, it's an isolated part made in a lab. When you read a study about food, you are reading about altered food not real food.

The sad truth is that most people, including researchers, do not take into consideration that when you alter a food, you alter its chemical composition. When the chemical composition changes, the effect it will have on the body changes. Research on altered food and research on vitamins made in a lab is not true nutrition research. It is research on the effects of altered food and the effects of lab-made vitamins on your health—that is all. It actually gives us no information about actual real food and your health.

But do not despair. Great research on the important role nutrition plays in your health does exist; to find it, you just have to look back to a time when unaltered food was readily available, which means prior to the 1960s.

Dr. Pottenger, Dr. Price, and Dr. Royal Lee were a few of the pioneers in whole food research.

However, there is another reason as to why research is not being done today on the effects of food and our health. The unfortunate truth is there is no money to be made by doing it. The fact is that money pays for research, and research money comes from investors hoping to make money. Whole food cannot be patented, and hence is not a source for profit. There is no one willing to pay for whole food research.

Once in a while, you will hear about a study on nutrition. When you do, look at it closely. Consider the source and dig deeper to find the types of foods or supplements that were tested. I encourage you not to just stop at the headline and assume what you are reading applies to whole food.

If you are interested in reading more of the research that was done on whole food prior to food being altered, visit the International Foundation for Nutrition and Health's website, or search on the Internet for some of the names mentioned above. You will be entering a fascinating world that looks back on how things used to be and how I believe they can be again, at least in your body.

END NOTES

1. Oxford Advanced Learner's Dictionary, s.v. "vitamin," accessed August 27, 2015, http://oxforddictionaries.com/us/definition/american_english/vitamin

2. IFIC Foundation, "Is Food Fortification Necessary? A Historical Perspective," *Food Insight Newsletter*, June 20, 2014, last modified June 24 2014, accessed August 27, 2015, http://www.foodinsight.org/Newsletter/Detail.aspx%3Ftopic%3DIs_ Food_Fortification_Necessary_A_Historical_Perspective#sthash. kN3Ft0Pe.dpuf

3. "What Is a Vitamin?" accessed September 1, 2015, http://www. drroyallee.com/the_truth_about_vitamins.html

4. Paul A. Offit "Don't Take Your Vitamins," *The New York Times*, June 8, 2013, accessed August 27, 2015, http://www.nytimes. com/2013/06/09/opinion/sunday/dont-take-your-vitamins. html?pagewanted=all&_r=0

5. E. R. Miller III, R. Pastor-Barriuso, D. Dalal, R. A. Riemersma, L. J. Appel, and E. Guallarhttp, "Meta-Analysis: High-Dosage Vitamin E Supplementation May Increase All-Cause Mortality," *Annals of Internal Medicine* 142, no. 1 (January 2005): 37-46, accessed September 1, 2015, http://annals.org/article.aspx?articleid=718097

6. Quoted in U.S. EPA Methyl Bromide Alternative Case Study Part of EPA 430-R-96-021, Case Studies, Volume 2, December 1996. Available on http://mbao.org/sulfury2.html

7. Albert W. Burgstahler, "Residual Fluoride In Food Fumigated With Sulfuryl Fluoride," Fluoride 38, no. 3(2005): 175-177, accessed September 1, 2015, http://www.fluorideresearch.org/383/ files/383175-177.pdf

8. EPA, "EPA Proposes to Withdraw Sulfuryl Fluoride Tolerances," para. 1, last modified March 31, 2015, accessed September 1, 2015, http://www.epa.gov/pesticides/sulfuryl-fluoride/evaluations.html

9. Ibid, para. 11.

10. Joseph M. Mercola, "Fluoride Hardens Your Arteries - Odds Are 6 in 10 You're Consuming This Poison Ingredient Daily," May 21, 2012, accessed August 27, 2015,http://articles.mercola.com/sites/ articles/archive/2012/05/21/fluoride-health-hazards.aspx

11. Phyllis J. Mullenix, "A New Perspective on Metals and Other Contaminants in Fluoridation Chemicals," *International Journal of Occupational and Environmental Health* 20, no. 2 (2014): 157-166, accessed August 27, 2015, http://momsagainstfluoridation.org/sites/ default/files/Mullenix%202014-2-2.pdf

12. Urvashi Rangan, "U.S. Department of Agriculture guts national organic law, September 19, 2013, accessed August 27, 2015, https://consumersunion.org/news/u-s-department-of-agriculture-guts-national-organic-law/

13. Stephanie Strom, "Lawsuit Challenges U.S.D.A. Rule Change on Organic Farming," New York Times, April 7, 2015, accessed August 27, 2015, http://www.nytimes.com/2015/04/08/business/lawsuit-challenges-change-in-rules-on-organic-farming.html?_r=0

14. Environmental Working Group, "Decoding Meat + Dairy Product Labels," 2011, accessed August 27, 2015, http://www.ewg.org/meateatersguide/decoding-meat-dairy-product-labels/#sthash.wGi2L9Bg.dpuf?

15. Ibid.

16. FDA, "What is the meaning of 'natural' on the label of food?" accessed August 27, 2015, http://www.fda.gov/aboutfda/transparency/basics/ucm214868.htm

CHAPTER 6

How to Recognize, Find, and Eat Food

"The assumption that human technology could improve on the wisdom of Nature has become a primary cause of disease in the modern world. We dissect food, take out the most glaringly obvious parts, attempt to recreate them in a laboratory, and label them as "active ingredients." In fact, it is the symphony of nutrients working synergistically that provides the quantum healing power of whole foods."
—Patrick Quillan, PhD, *American Journal of Natural Medicine*, September 2002

Nature Is Smarter Than We Are

We've spent some time talking about how the body works, why most of what we eat falls under my definition of C.R.A.P, chemically-ridden altered products, and why that's a problem for our bodies. I hope you're beginning to understand that if your goal is good health, perfect weight, and a long vital life, your current food choices will not support you in reaching that goal. Some of you may be thinking, *I eat three meals a day and include all the five food groups—so this information must not apply to me.*

Unfortunately, that may not be true. If you are not making conscious choices about where you shop for food and how you prepare what you purchase, chances are at least a portion of what you're eating is C.R.A.P. and does not meet the definition of food, or the needs of your body.

So are you ready? Have you been saturated enough with what is wrong? Are you ready for some solutions?

You may be wondering how to find food if you cannot trust the labels and if everything has chemicals added to it. Actually, it is easier than you may think. Eating real food comes down to two things: how it's grown and how it's prepared. It really is that simple.

And simple takes us back to simpler times. Think about the way your great-grandparents used to get and prepare their food. And no, you don't have to have been there to know or worry about having to grow your own vegetables and raise your own cows. Although, if you were so inclined to, it would certainly ensure you will be doing a good deed for your body.

Fortunately, there are more convenient ways. But before we start to look at food itself, let's start with a few basic principles that will help you identify food and avoid problems that some foods can cause you.

Nature is smarter than we are. I have yet to find a human-designed anything that is better and works more efficiently or longer without negative effects than what is designed by natural law.

The fact is that everything humans require for optimal health is found in food. Real food! Not the stuff you find in a box on the shelf in your supermarket, but food the way nature made it.

I operate under the premise that nature and the human body are naturally in harmony with one another. So when making choices about what my body needs, I ask three simple questions:

1. Is the food in alignment with nature? In other words, is it grown or raised naturally?
2. Would people I consider healthy consume this product?
3. Have humans been consuming this product for more than a generation? What are the effects it's had on their offspring?

If I cannot answer yes to all three, then it does not pass my criteria for something I will put in my body.

I remember when the alkaline water craze started. I asked myself, "Is drinking alkaline water in line with what nature does?"

Natural spring water generally has a pH of 7.5. So, NO, since alkaline water has a pH of 8.5 or higher, it is, therefore, not in alignment with nature.

Would my healthy friends consume it? YES, they were all doing it and claiming it was the best thing ever!

Have humans on a large scale been doing it for more than a generation? NO.

So alkaline water was a NO for me.

It wasn't long before I started seeing cases of ill health in my office that I traced back to drinking alkaline water.

One such case was a pregnant mom who was drinking alkaline water to counter her acid reflux. When she came to see me, she had just gotten out of the hospital for kidney stones where she had required morphine for pain. Yes—I did say she was pregnant.

When I looked at her blood, I found she was also anemic. Anemia and pregnancy are not an ideal combination. We changed her water, gave her digestive support to help her acid reflux, and supported her for anemia. Several weeks later, we reran her blood test to see how her anemia was doing. I am happy to say she was no longer anemic, and we had to cut back on the supplements she was taking because her iron levels were so good.

Just like the distilled water craze of the 80s, which was proven to be problematic because it leached minerals out of the body, alkaline water has shown to be problematic for a couple of reasons.

1. It hinders proper digestion and absorption of food by creating too high of a pH in the stomach thus interfering with absorption of minerals and the entire digestive process.
2. Because of the excess of non-absorbable minerals that end up as sediment in the kidneys, it predisposes people to developing kidney stones.

I have seen many well-intentioned people do things that end up harming them. You may think me old-fashioned, but I also know I will not be doing harm to others or myself by recommending fads that are later proven harmful. This is the principle I used to heal my own body and this is the principle I have used with my clients for over 15 years…because it works.

Food Preparation: Phytic Acid

One of the things about food that has been lost in our hurry-up-and-eat- now world, pointing back to the "old-fashioned ways," is the art of food preparation. In order for certain foods to be nutritious, they need to be prepared prior to eating. Soybeans, for instance, are basically indigestible, unless fermented. Hence, the reason traditionally the Chinese and Japanese ate tofu, tempeh, and soy sauce instead of soybeans, or soy flour, etc. In their nonfermented form, soybeans contain a substance that hinders digestion. Eating soybeans unfermented can cause gas bloating and digestive distress, as well as block the absorption of minerals, all not good things. This is why food preparation matters. Classically, foods were prepared in ways that supported digestion, but today, we have abandoned this art.

This is important for you to understand because I do not want you to spend lots of time and money making dietary changes, only to be losing the benefits because you are eating food in a form that hinders digestion.

So what's this substance that makes soybeans indigestible if not fermented? It is called phytic acid, and phytic acid is not just in soybeans, it is in lots of the foods we eat. Phytic acid is in grains, nuts, seeds, and beans.

According to Weston Price foundation, a foundation dedicated to promoting whole food consumption,

> *"Phytic acid not only grabs on to or chelates important minerals, but also inhibits enzymes that we need to digest our food."*

How and why does it do this? It does this because it is doing its job. Phytic acid is in plants to inhibit the seed from germinating under the wrong conditions. If a seed germinates at the wrong time, i.e., a time when the conditions are not good for survival, then it will likely die (not a good thing). Phytic acid stays active, inhibiting the enzymes that promote germination until the conditions are right for growth. Enzymes are substances that are needed to activate every chemical process in the body. If enzymes are inhibited, then chemical reactions cannot happen and digestion is inhibited. Ultimately, digestion can be looked at as one big chemical reaction.

Phytic acid is also a great binder. It will bind to metals and minerals at a high rate. It can actually be used in certain medical cases to clean the body of harmful substances, which can be a good thing; however, if you are eating food to get minerals, and phytic acid is binding to minerals and taking them out of your body, that is not a good thing.

Although phytic acid naturally occurs in food, classically, it has not been a problem for us in our diets. This is because traditional food preparation eliminated its effect. However, due to modern-day agriculture practices and the loss of our knowledge about proper food preparation, it now represents a problem for us.

Historically, grains and legumes were soaked, sprouted, fermented, and soured, as is the case with sourdough, prior to cooking, which eliminated the phytic acid.

We have lost the art of preparing our food to enhance nutrient density, and, in losing this, we unknowingly hindered our ability to absorb the nutrients that are in the food we are eating. Not only are there fewer minerals in our food due to how it is grown but now we are not able to absorb what is still there.

Sally Fallon's book, *Nourishing Traditions* does a good job of reeducating us about how to prepare foods for maximum health benefits. By sprouting and fermenting your food, you not only decrease phytic acid levels, which increase mineral absorption and enzyme activity but, in the case of fermenting, you can actually increase B vitamin concentration and probiotic intake, two things essential for a strong, healthy body.

The foods highest in phytic acid are unsprouted and unfermented grains such as found in breads and other flour products, unsoaked beans, nuts and seeds, and worst of all, because it is highest in phytic acid, nonfermented soy.[1,2]

Grain

Grains are a major part of the American diet. From wheat, oats, corn, and rice, the average person is estimated to eat around 200 pounds per year, and that amount has only increased over the years.[3]

Wheat is, by far, the highest consumed grain with an estimated 140 plus pounds making it into the average person's body each year. You know the great American diet of cereal for breakfast, followed by a sandwich for lunch, and pasta for dinner.

Have you ever eaten like that in a day? If you stop to think about what you consumed, it was mostly wheat! It had just been shaped into different forms often using chemicals to promote the desired shape.

As I mentioned earlier, wheat and grain in general has been a major player in the human diet for thousands of years. And grains can have many nutritious benefits. When eaten in their whole food form, they are high in B vitamins, rich in minerals, provide a good source of fiber, and even some essential fatty acids. Grains, when eaten in combination can also provide the complete amino acid profile the human body needs. Grains also digest in a way that, when eaten in small portions, help keep your blood sugar balanced. They have even been shown to be cancer protective—all in all a good thing.

However, we have never eaten them in quantities like we do today. Humans are omnivores, which means our digestive tract is built to digest small amounts of a variety of foods. If we were meant to eat large quantities of grains then our digestive tract would look more like a camel's with four chambers in our stomach to properly break down the all-plant diet. However, we have just one chamber designed to eat small amounts of a variety of foods.

C.R.A.P. Form of Grain

A lot has been already said about the altering of grain. To recap, In general, the grains we are eating in this country have had lots of chemicals added to them in the form of synthetic fertilizers, pesticides, and weed controllers while being grown. As mentioned in the chapter on gluten, wheat, the grain we are eating the most of, has been hybridized so much the genetic structure of the seeds barely resemble those of the past.[4]

It is also harvested in ways that strips away the germ and the bran, removing most of the vitamins, healthy fats, and healthy fiber. Before it even leaves the farm, it is chemically ridden and has been significantly altered from its original state, leaving the starchy endosperm, which breaks down into sugar in the body.

From there it goes to the manufacturer, where, more often than not, chemicals (including potassium bromate, benzoyl peroxide, even chlorine gas) are added to it in an attempt to make it have a longer shelf life, look whiter, and taste like something you want to eat. (The use of chemicals to whiten flour is banned in England and many other countries. Not here.)[5]

Here they are used in massive amounts. Several sources link bleached flour to diabetes. During the bleaching process, a chemical called Alloxan is produced. This chemical is used in labs to make lab rats diabetic for research purposes. It is known to destroy the pancreatic cells that make insulin.[6, 7]

Is the increase in diabetes linked to flour bleaching?

I think this is a very good question. Some professionals say yes, some say there isn't enough evidence. But is eating white flour really worth the risk?

Then, in an attempt to add back in a bit of the nutrition that has been lost, synthetic vitamins are thrown in. They are added because, prior to doing so, people where developing B deficiency diseases from the lack of vitamins in the bread they were eating.

What a mess.

So, why play with fire? Why feed your family and yourself something that is devoid of nutrition, has chemicals added that are banned for use in other countries, and could potentially be killing off pancreas cells? And adding extra glucose to your body is probably making you fat.

Now perhaps you are thinking you are safe if you only eat organic whole grain. That's a great start but, unfortunately, not enough. Because most people rarely properly prepare grains prior to cooking them, we often don't get the benefit from eating them that we should.

As stated in Sally Fallon's cookbook *Nourishing Traditions*, "Our ancestors and virtually all pre-industrialized peoples, soaked or fermented their grains prior to making them into porridge, breads, cakes, and casseroles."

If not properly soaked and/or fermented, grain, because of its phytic acid levels, can hinder digestion and leach minerals from your body. It can actually take nutrition away from you. For this reason, I call white flour and white sugar negative foods because you are actually less nourished after you eat them than you were before.

Although the need to properly prepare grain is true of all grains, it is especially true of wheat because it is such a major part of what we eat in this country.

So what did you really have for breakfast, lunch, and dinner? You had a grain that now fits the definition of C.R.A.P. better than it does food. You are eating the shell of what was once wheat.

Food Form of Grain

I know that bread tastes so good, and, for many people I have talked to, they would rather suffer the consequences than give it up. However, perhaps you do not have to choose between your health and your taste buds. Have your bread and pasta, but see if you can find some that has been soured and is freshly made. If you are not able to, then use pasta and breads as placeholders instead of as your meal. Have a piece of toast or a small amount of pasta and add to it what will be your nutrition for that meal. Or, better yet, learn to prepare your own. *Nourishing Traditions* does a good job of teaching you how to prepare grains, and gives you recipes.

If your digestion is functioning properly and can digest them, then having grains is a good choice, as there are nutrients in grain that you do not get from other foods. However, you must be eating them in their whole form and they must be prepared in a way to promote proper digestion and mineral absorption.

Remember, grains are very high in carbohydrates, so be careful about your portion size, or you may watch you waist size expand. You do not need to eat a lot of grains to meet your carbohydrate needs at a meal; just about ½ cup will do the trick. Avoid bleached flours always. And, if you are able to find freshly made bread, make sure it is fermented as found in sourdough.

C.R.A.P Grain	Food Form of Grain
✗ Flour over 3 days old	✓ Whole grain that has been minimally processed such as oat groats or brown rice
✗ Flour that has been bleached	✓ Grain that has been soaked prior to cooking
✗ Flour that has had the germ removed	✓ Grain that has been made into flour recently
✗ Grain that has been altered such as quick oats or white rice	✓ Grain that has been fermented such as sourdough

Nuts, Seeds and Legumes

Nuts, seeds, and legumes (or beans) can be a nice source of both protein and fats. They are also rich in minerals and high in fiber, and are a nice compliment to any diet. Nuts and seeds are a great on-the-go snack. Due to the balance of protein, fat, and carbohydrate, they are a great way to keep blood sugar levels balanced between meals. Legumes or beans are a great compliment to any diet since they can be precooked to have on hand for a quick meal of beans and rice with some avocado.

C.R.A.P. Form of Nuts, Seeds, and Legumes

Nuts that are cooked and salted and have sat around for a while are not good for you. The cooking turns the oils into free radicals (see the section on fats), the added salt is iodized chemical salt, and when they sit around the oil goes rancid.

Nuts are also high in phytic acid, and thus are best when consumed after they have been soaked in warm water or sprouted in the case of nuts. *Nourishing Traditions* also outlines how long is best to soak the various kinds of nuts, seed, and legumes.

Food Form of Nuts, Seeds & Legumes

If you are making a shake or other recipe calling for nuts make sure to soak them. If you are buying them at the store, make sure to buy raw or if they have them, raw sprouted. I recommend people who use nuts as a main protein source to make sure their nuts are soaked. However, if you are having nuts as a snack occasionally and soaked is not available, then eating them organic and raw is the next best thing.

Nuts are high in arginine. If you get cold sores or have the herpes virus in your system then be mindful of how many nuts you eat. Arginine promotes the replication of the virus. If you are getting outbreaks, then you may want to skip nuts for a while.

C.R.A.P. Nuts, Seeds & Beans	Food Form of Nuts, Seeds & Beans
✘ Nuts and seeds that are roasted	✔ Sprouted nuts
✘ Nuts that are old	✔ Soaked and freshly ground-up seeds
✘ Beans from a can	✔ Organic, raw nut butters in an air-tight glass jar
✘ Unsoaked beans	✔ Beans soaked prior to cooking
✘ Nuts, seeds, and beans that have been ground-up and exposed to the air	✔ Homemade nut butters
✘ Ground flax seeds 14 hours or older	
✘ Roasted nut butters	
✘ Nut butters in plastic	

Soy: The Four Strikes Against It!

I rarely advise that one single food be eliminated from your diet completely. In fact, generally speaking, I believe a person's diet should include a wide variety of foods, particularly foods that are personal favorites. However, when it comes to soy, I'm singing another tune.

I have nothing against soy itself. In the past, it has certainly been a food that had health benefits when consumed in small amounts, particularly in its fermented form. If I'd been in practice 50 years ago, I would have probably said soy was a great adjunctive food. I would have likely promoted the consumption of small amounts of fermented soy, particularly if you were a woman with declining estrogen levels. However, today is a very different environment than 50 years ago, and soy is a very different food. So, for the most part, I put almost all soy on the C.R.A.P. list.

Strike 1: Hello, Belly Bloat and Osteoporosis!

As mentioned, soy is very high in phytic acid. Phytic acid can block the activation of digestive enzymes, which can interfere with your digestive process, leading to bloating, distention, and gas, among other health issues.

Also, phytic acid can bind to minerals, and eating too much over time can create mineral deficiency diseases such as osteoporosis and anemia. Soy has more phytic acid than most other foods, so it is a particularly bad offender in these two areas.

Strike 2: Can you say guinea pig?

Soy is one of the most widely genetically modified (GMO) crops. Ninety percent of crops sold in this country are grown from genetically modified seeds. As mentioned, GMO food is way too new and unstudied to take the risk of being the guinea pigs for big business.

And be warned…in today's food model, highly processed non-fermented forms of soy are in almost everything!

Strike 3: The Bean without a Conscience

If a plant could have a personality, the soy of today would definitely be a sketchy figure, lacking in some essential morals. The soybean industry is responsible for many crimes against the earth and against fellow farmers.

The main company that owns the patent on the GMO soy seed approved in this country spends millions of dollars a year suing small farmers out of business. So, when you buy soybeans, you are supporting their unscrupulous practices.

Soybean farmers enjoy massive subsidies, a reported $27.8 billion from 1995-2012. There is a lot of controversy about the benefits versus detriments to this level of subsidy and many would argue that it does a lot more harm than good, especially since the majority of subsidies go to a small minority of large-scale GMO growing farmers.

Add to that the fact that soy farming is also responsible for massive amounts of deforestation across the globe and you have some pretty compelling reasons to avoid soy. By saying no to soy, you are saying no to these highly questionable and environmentally damaging practices.

Strike 4: The Major Reason I Say No to Soy

Soy promotes estrogen production. I hear you, "What's wrong with that?" Particularly if you are a perimenopausal or menopausal woman hot flashing all over the place. Wouldn't a little support with estrogen be good? In theory, yes; however, there is one problem that gets in the way of this being true and it is called xenoestrogens. These are chemicals that *act* like estrogens in the body but aren't. Exposure to these chemicals is creating what *feels* like an epidemic of estrogen dominance, a state of having too much estrogen in relation to other hormones. When this important relationship is out of balance, we become predisposed to developing all kinds of diseases.

In women, estrogen dominance increases the chances of developing breast cancer, uterine fibroids, and ovarian cancer. In men, it increases the chances of developing breast cancer, infertility, and gynecomastia, the developing of man boobs. Not to be confused with regular fat, it is the development of actual breast tissue. And, worst of all, studies have shown that in little boys xenoestrogens are responsible for smaller genital size and increased effeminate behavior.[8]

In addition, studies also show it is becoming common for girls to start puberty earlier; one of the main theories for this is the massive amount of estrogen exposure. Because of the predominance of this problem, scientists are now recommending that girls "should be evaluated (for health problems) if this [breast development] occurs before age 7 in white girls and before age 6 in African-American girls," as opposed to the previous recommendation of age 8.[9]

So what does this have to do with soy? Soy stimulates the production of estrogen by keeping the receptor sites in the "on" position longer. When estrogen production is increased, estrogen dominance and the problems associated with it can be exacerbated. It has been my experience that many of the clients I see are experiencing some form of estrogen dominance.

And if an increased risk of diseases like cancer and uterine fibroids isn't enough; too much estrogen promotes the storage of fat. This is why women's bodies have a lot more rounded areas than most men have. With an estimated 68% of Americans being overweight and obesity at well over 35%, the last thing we need to do in the country is promote fat storage!

So I say **No to Soy** in almost all cases except just a few in very small amounts! If soy is fermented, as is the case with tempeh, then the phytic acid has been neutralized and the risk of it impeding digestion and robbing your body of the benefits of the minerals in your food has been minimized. Be careful you aren't spending all your time, energy, and money on making positive dietary changes only to lose the benefit of the nutrient dense food because edamame is your favorite appetizer.

C.R.A.P. Soy	Food Form of Soy
✗ All nonorganic soy (is probably GMO soy)	✓ Organic fermented soy
✗ All nonfermented soy	✓ Tempeh, tofu in small amounts
✗ Edamame	✓ Gluten-free organic soy sauce
✗ Soy protein powders	✓ Nama shoy yu
✗ Soy food additives	✓ Gluten-free tamari
✗ Soy oil	
✗ Vegetable oils (most contain soy oil)	

Fruits and Veggies

Vegetables are a major source of our vitamins and minerals; so, regardless of whether you and/or your children like them, they are an essential part of a nutritious diet.

The easiest way to get vegetables to be a part of your family's regular diet is to start children out eating vegetables from the very beginning. When you first introduce food to little ones, introduce greens even before you introduce sweet foods like banana. That way, their palate will develop around the more bitter flavor of green vegetables.

Increasing vegetable intake is necessary for almost all the people I see. For your children, whose palates are already formed, my best suggestion is get on the computer and look up clever ways to get your kids to eat vegetables. Some kids love shakes, and that's an easy way to hide green things. Some parents suggest blending veggies into their pasta sauces, and some make homemade Jello cubes and incorporate veggies into them.

To help you add veggies to your diet refer to the chart "making friends with vegetables" on the following pages. Exploring your likes and dislikes in the vegetable kingdom can be fun, and once you start eating real organic foods with more flavor, you may just find out that you actually like them. Regardless of how you feel about them, I guarantee your body will love you for adding more in.

C.R.A.P. Form of Fruits and Vegetables

Yep, even fruits and vegetables can fall under the C.R.A.P. category. Now do not get me wrong—on a gradient, you're way better off eating any kind of vegetable than you are eating any kind of white processed flour product; but, that said, it is important to know that not all fruits and veggies are created equal. Due to changes in agricultural practices that I've already discussed, fruits and vegetables have the potential to be sorely lacking in nutrients and loaded with chemicals. Especially commercially grown ones.

One of my favorite admissions of the difference between commercially grown and organically grown fruits and veggies was an ad I saw sponsored by several of the major supermarkets.

It came out around the time they first started selling organic. In the ad, there is a photo of the produce section in a typical American supermarket. The picture showed a large produce section with a small square of vegetables in the middle labeled organic produce. It then went on to explain all the reasons organic was better for you.

"Studies have found significantly higher levels of vitamins, minerals, and cancer-fighting antioxidants in organic produce," it touted.

It went on to say, "Because of the higher nutrient levels, eating organically grown fruits and vegetables can reduce your risk of chronic disease and lessen your need for dietary supplements."

And then my favorite,

"Clean" rich soil, where organic produce comes from, also creates rich flavors. So you don't just get better nutrition from organic food, you get better taste."

In other words, they are telling you all the reasons why the majority of the produce in their store was not as good for you and lacked in flavor as compared to their organic counterpart. Even the major sellers of commercially grown produce know there is a difference.

Food Form of Fruits and Vegetables

Be sure you are getting what you are paying more for, make sure you are buying food that is raised according to the true organic laws. Also, make sure you are eating them in season and picked fresh.

To do this, just head back to your farmers market, or get your produce delivered from a local CSA (consumer-supported agriculture). If those options are not available to you, buy from a small health food store that sources their food locally.

When buying your produce from these kinds of sellers, you can talk to the people who have a direct relationship to the food and ask them how the food is grown.

Not all growers are certified organic, even though they may grow using the practices of true sustainable farming. The cost and paperwork to become certified is often prohibitive for small farmers. When you talk to them directly, you can find out how they grow their food. My experience is that people who are committed to farming in sustainable ways are *into* their food and are happy to talk with you about it.

One other point I need to mention is to watch your fruit to vegetable ratio. I was just working with a woman a few weeks ago who ate well, exercised every day, yet was gaining weight. I had her follow The 21-Day Diet Detox so we could identify if the reason she was not losing weight was a hormonal issue or a lifestyle issue.

After a week on the program, she came in and she had not lost a pound. I looked at her diet record and saw that she was eating much more fruit than was recommended. I suggested we adjust her intake of fruit and see what happened. She came back a week later and had lost 5 pounds. For her, the extra fruit was enough to push her body into fat storing instead of fat burning mode. It only takes 1 tablespoon of honey, or 1 whole banana to almost reach your meal's carbohydrate needs. So pay attention.

To balance your food intake, you want to choose to eat at least ¾ vegetables to no more than ¼ fruit. And not just any fruit; make sure the fruit you choose is lower in sugar. Too much sugar, as my client above experienced can cause problems, even when it is coming from fruit.

So, yes, eat organic fruit, just choose what are known as low-glycemic fruits (fruit that breakdown slower and thereby enter the blood stream slower) and the keep the amount in check.

Organic Low-Glycemic Fruit

Organic Low-Glycemic Fruit

Avocado

Green-tipped Banana

Blackberries

Blueberries

Cherries

Cranberries (unsweetened)

Fuji or green apple

Red Grapes

Lemons

Limes

Papaya

Peach

Pear

Plum

Pomegranate

Raspberries

Strawberries

C.R.A.P. Vegetables & Fruit	Food Form of Vegetables and Fruit
✗ Grown using pesticides & herbicides	✓ Grown according to 1990 organic standards
✗ Grown far away and shipped	✓ Grown using sustainable agriculture practices
✗ Non-organic commercially farmed	✓ Grown locally
✗ Grown using glyphosates	✓ Picked ripe
✗ Picked green	✓ Eaten while still fresh
✗ Sprayed with preservatives and synthetic waxes	✓ Low-glycemic fruits
✗ Canned anything	

Dairy: Milk and Milk Products

When we speak of dairy, we are talking about everything that is made from the milk of an animal—eggs are not in the category. This is a question I am asked often, and, since eggs are often sold in the dairy section of the supermarket, it is easy to see where the confusion comes from.

As I mentioned earlier, my medical training is based in Chinese medicine. I love this medicine for many reasons; however, one of my favorite things I learned from studying it is the understanding that food or any other substance can have varying effects on the body.

The practice of Chinese Herbal Medicine was developed over thousands of years. Its foundation comes from the observation of how food and herbs affect the body and is categorized in the following ways: will the substance promote dryness, or promote fluid production; add warmth, or add coolness. That information can then be used to assess how to eat in a way that balances the body.

For example, often skin problems have a heat component to them. So it is recommended that warming foods be avoided. Knowing this can be very helpful when dealing with a health challenge. In China, you may still be able to go to an herbalist, get assessed, and be given a prescription, not for herbal medicine but for dinner. Then you would walk to the restaurant next door and eat a meal prepared for you based on your doctor's prescription.

Paul Pitchford in his book, *Healing With Whole Food* makes this ancient knowledge available to the public and I think it is a great read for anyone interested in learning more about food.

In the Chinese food system, dairy is identified as building fluids in the body. This is great if you are a person who is very dry as can be the case with the elderly. However, if you are a person who tends to get phlegmy, or if you have a cold or flu and are experiencing lots of mucous, it's not so good, as it will promote mucous production.

These properties noticed about milk are from milk that is in its natural state; however, the majority of milk sold in this country has been altered.

C.R.A.P. Form of Dairy

There is no type of food that I have seen a more dramatic shift from food to C.R.A.P. than in dairy. The way in which cows are raised in commercial dairies and the hormones and chemicals used to keep the cows producing milk nonstop 365 days a year, combined with the way dairy is processed, have changed the dairy we eat here in America from something that was once a nutritious food to a real potential health hazard.

The changes made to dairy, not only enhance its mucous-promoting tendency, they also do a lot of other things that end up making dairy problematic. I would say that next to gluten, dairy is the number one intolerance I identify in my clients.

When you pasteurize milk, heat it to high temperature to kill off all bacteria, you are not only killing potential toxic bacteria but you are also killing all the beneficial bacteria that naturally occur in milk. If you take a raw cream and let it sit on the counter the naturally occurring bacteria will sour it and turn it into sour cream. It is quite edible. However, if you leave pasteurized milk on the counter it will rot and likely make you sick if you drank it. Why is that? That is because the naturally occurring bacteria will not allow pathogenic bacteria to grow. However, if the naturally occurring bacteria are not present then pathogenic bacteria take up residence and will grow exclusively.

Pasteurizing milk also destroys the naturally occurring enzymes that help you absorb the calcium in it, making what was once a rich calcium source a very poor one. Remember, just because the vitamins or minerals are there in what you are eating doesn't mean your body can absorb them. Pasteurizing also destroys the fat-soluble vitamins such as vitamin A and D, hence the reason milk is enriched with those vitamins.

Pasteurizing also destroys the enzymes that help you process lactose, thus creating lactose intolerance. To make matters worse, we often remove the fat from the milk. I was taught that in order to digest milk protein, you need milk fat. So without the fat, you are now unable to properly absorb the protein.

Then the milk is homogenized, pushed through a sieve to breakdown the particle into very small units. This keeps the milk from separating. Remember when I talked about leaky gut. With the smaller particle sizes created by homogenization it becomes easier for those particles to get into the blood stream, thereby making the development of a food intolerance much more likely.

What was once a food rich in calcium, vitamin A & D, healthy fat and protein is now a substance with the fat and fat soluble vitamins missing, the protein and calcium indigestible, a lot of lactose you cannot breakdown, and a very high potential for causing a food intolerance.

If that isn't bad enough, substances like carrageenan and other chemicals are added to replace the thickness lost when the fat is removed. Carrageenan is implicated in causing inflammatory bowel diseases such as Crohn's disease and ulcerative colitis.

I was the milk girl on TV for over 5 years and yet I couldn't even drink the stuff; it upset my stomach too much. When we shot the commercial, I had to spit the milk out after each take.

I know your head is probably spinning right now. If you are like most people, you probably thought dairy products were really, really good for you, loaded with calcium and protein.

Well, actually, you are correct for some dairy. Real dairy is all of that; you have just not been eating real dairy.

Food Sources of Dairy

So how can you find real dairy? Eat your dairy in its raw form. This solves all of the problems. You get your fat-soluble vitamins, your calcium and proteins are absorbable, and the lactase is still working, so you will break down the lactose. Problem solved!

Now some people will go online and read about raw dairy and be scared by what they read. I get it. There is a lot of information that is against raw dairy. There is a big interest in shutting raw dairies down. In many states, they have succeeded in making the sale of raw dairy illegal.

Fortunately, in California, we can still get it. However, the battle is ongoing. Why would this be happening? If you ask yourself a simple question, you may come to your own conclusion. They pasteurize milk to kill off pathogenic bugs. Where are those bugs coming from? Why would the milk have pathogenic bugs in the first place? Perhaps because the cows are living in unsanitary conditions, hooked up to milking machines 24/7.

It is true that in order to produce clean milk, your cows have to be healthy and live in clean uncrowded conditions. Pasteurized or not, why would you want to drink milk from sick cows that are living in toxic environments? Raw milk cows, however, have to be raised in a very clean environment, and in California, at least, are highly monitored by the USDA.

However, if you are concerned at all about drinking raw milk, then just do not drink it, but also do not drink pasteurized. Just skip milk all together.

Do not worry about where you are going to get your calcium, you can replace your milk with one of the milk substitutes, like hemp or almond milk; if you buy them in the store, they are fortified just like the milk you are drinking is. Truthfully, you should be getting your calcium from calcium rich vegetables, like collard greens, kale, turnip greens, spinach, sun dried tomatoes, and okra, alfalfa, and skip the fortified foods altogether.

Regardless of whether you choose to drink raw milk, by all means, eat raw cheese. There is little debate about the safety of raw cheese, so eat your cheese in its raw form. Make sure your children are eating cheese in its raw form as well. Dairy intolerance is so prevalent in children; you do not want to take a chance of them developing it by feeding them pasteurized dairy.

Raw cheese does not taste different than pasteurized cheese. It is not the pasteurization that determines the flavor, but rather how the cheese is made. If you do not like the taste of one, just try another.

All yogurt is pasteurized in California. When they test for bacteria it is impossible to quickly test the difference between the healthy bacteria found in yogurt verse pathogenic bacteria, so the government in this state does not allow raw yogurt to be sold. In some cases, people tolerate yogurt even though it is not raw because the added bacteria help digest the milk and make it less of a problem. If you are a person who loves yogurt, then make sure you are eating yogurt with no sugar added, one with real living healthy bacteria in it, and, of course, is organic and whole fat. Many people also tolerate goat and sheep dairy much better than cow because they have been exposed less over their lifetime. You might try eating only those in small amounts and see how you feel.

Everyone is different, so see for yourself how your body handles dairy. After following The 21-Day Diet Detox you will have an opportunity to see if dairy is negatively affecting you. If you have allergies, sinus congestion, skin rashes, a digestive problem or any health issue that improves while on the program, a dairy intolerance may be part of your problem. When you add raw dairy back in after the 3-week pause, pay close attention. If your symptoms return or increase, keep it out entirely for at least 3 months, and then try adding back the raw form again and see how you feel. If you get symptoms again, then it would be a good idea to choose to keep it out permanently. It will be of great help to your health.

C.R.A.P. Dairy	Food Form of Dairy
✗ Pasteurized milk and milk products	✓ Raw milk and milk products
✗ Homogenized milk and milk products	✓ Raw cheese
✗ Non-fat milk and milk products	✓ Organic whole milk yogurt
✗ Low-fat milk and milk products	✓ Raw whole cream
✗ Milk products from cows raised on feed lots	✓ Raw whole milk
✗ Milk products from cows raised on RBST	✓ Milk from locally raised animals
✗ Milk products from cows raised with antibiotics	✓ Milk Alternatives: home-made almond, macadamia, cashew, or other nut milk
	✓ Raw butter or butter from grass-fed pasture-raised cows

Meat

"How can you expect to stay healthy if what you are eating to promote that health is sick?"—C.S.

Twenty percent of the human body is made up of protein. Protein plays a crucial role in almost all biological processes, and amino acids are the building blocks of protein. The body takes protein from the food you eat, breaks it down into individual amino acids, and then reassembles the amino acids into new proteins.

A large proportion of our cells, muscles, and tissue are made up of amino acids. Amino acids are essential for all-important bodily functions because they are what enzymes are made from and enzymes play a key role in the breakdown, transport, and the storage of all nutrients. Amino acids have an influence on the function of all your organs, glands, tendons, and arteries. They are essential for healing wounds and repairing tissue, especially in the muscles, bones, skin, and hair as well as playing an important role in detoxification.

They are also important for a healthy balanced brain. Amino acids play an essential role in the formation of the brain neurotransmitters. Neurotransmitters, the chemicals in the brain that affect your mood, are made from amino acids. The amino acid, L-tryptophane, for example, is partly what melatonin, the neurotransmitter that supports sleep, is made from.

Every day, the body needs amino acids. The body can manufacture and synthesize some amino acids on its own. Others, however, known as essential amino acids, have to be supplied from the food you eat.

In your body, at any given time, there is an available pool of free amino acids. This pool is replenished when the protein eaten is broken down in the gastrointestinal tract into the individual amino acids. Once broken down, they can be put back together as new proteins. The entire amino acid pool is used up and replaced three to four times a day.[10]

This means that the body has to be supplied with new essential amino acids every day. When we are under stress, doing a lot of detoxifying, and/or healing, or exercising a lot, the protein needs of the body go up.

Protein is found in many food sources—vegetables, grains, legumes, and meat alike. However, most sources such as vegetables, grains, and legumes only contain a portion of the essential amino acids needed. To replenish your amino acid profile from those sources, pay attention to what you are eating and eat a variety of foods that contain all of the essential amino acids. Meat, fish, and eggs, however, are complete protein sources. They contain all of the necessary amino acids, making them an easy source of protein.

Before I say my next piece, and I start to rile a few of you, let me start by saying I was a vegetarian for many, many years. I love the idea of a vegetarian lifestyle. It is in alignment with my personal choice preferences. That said, I have met very few people leading fast-paced, stress-filled lives who are able to sustain their health long term while on a vegetarian or vegan diet.

From my observation, if you have a low-stress life and can spend the time to cook your own food, are willing to eat lots of vegetables, and whole, properly prepared grains and beans, instead of packaged vegetarian food, then a vegetarian or vegan diet is a great diet choice.

However, if your life is busy, you are on the go a lot, and under stress, or if you have any digestive difficulties, this may not be the time to be a vegetarian or vegan. It is just too difficult to get all the amino acids you need, and protein is way too important to be missing out on.

C.R.A.P. It's Even in Your Meat.

Yep, even the meat sold in the store fits the definition of C.R.A.P.

Meat over the years, especially red meat and meat fat has been blamed for several health problems. It is implicated in causing heart disease. It is blamed for causing cancer. It is blamed for causing inflammation.

But I am not convinced that it is really meat itself that is causing all of these things, but rather the large quantities of sick, polluted meat that people are eating; that is the problem. Because meat contains fat, and toxins stick to fat, meat that is not well raised can contain a lot of chemicals and excess hormones, a real problem for your health.

Unfortunately, if you are not paying close attention to where your meat is coming from, then it is **not** well raised, and I can assure you it has chemicals and excess hormones in it.

In this country, we have decided that it is perfectly fine to raise animals in ways that have nothing to do with raising a healthy animal. We feed them food that is not part of their natural diet. Cows, for instance, do not have a digestive tract that was designed to eat grain. Their digestive tract is designed to digest grass. When you feed cows grain, they develop a gut infection of a particular strain of E. coli, which is not normally found in their system. That form of E. coli happens to not only be pathogenic to the cow, but also deadly to humans.[11]

And yet most of the cattle in this country are raised on grain. The choice to feed cows grain supports the grower because it quickly fattens cows up, but creates a whole host of other problems, some of which we will discuss a bit further on.

Most, if not all, commercially raised animals are also raised in what are called CAFOs, confined animal feeding operations. According to the EPA website, CAFOs *"congregate animals, feed, manure and urine, dead animals, and production operations on a small land area. Feed is brought to the animals rather than the animals grazing or otherwise seeking feed in pastures, fields, or on rangeland."*[12] Sounds lovely, doesn't it?

To make it worse, large CAFOs can house more than 50,000 animals in this way.

When animals are raised in close confinement like this, they are more prone to infection. The high stress created by their living conditions weakens their immunity. Combine this with the unsanitary conditions they live in, which makes infections common. Because of this, antibiotics are needed often.

Antibiotics are also used to promote weight gain in these animals. This is being blamed for creating antibiotic-resistant bacteria, and is a health problem for those of us who then eat the antibiotics in the meat.

Hormones have been used for decades in the meat and dairy industries. Hormones make animals gain weight faster. More weight means more meat, which means more profit for the producer. Synthetic estrogens and testosterone and growth hormones are the most common hormones used in meat. These practices used on a large scale here in the United States are outlawed in many European countries.

According to the website WebMD.com, "How much hormone is in a hamburger, and could it hurt you? The answer is, no one really knows. Studies show the added hormones do show up in beef and milk, pushing their estrogen and testosterone content to the high end of normal for cows. Whether that translates to increased risk for humans is the question."[13]

So, here we go again, we are back to the old guinea pig factor "Not sure, but let's keep using them until someone can prove they are bad." But wait a minute. Do we really not know? We know that too much estrogen in a lifetime increases the risk of developing several cancers.[14]

If we are ingesting meat high in added hormones, doesn't that point towards a problem?

The problems continue when animals are sent to the slaughterhouse. It is required by law that animals are sent to FDA-approved slaughterhouses. This, in itself, is not bad, but, in this country, there is a monopoly on FDA-approved slaughterhouses, so an animal must travel long distances to get to one. This means a lot of time for the animal in very confined quarters. Which is, you guessed it, stressful to the animal. This increases the stress hormones in the meat.

Also, because the number of slaughterhouses is limited, they are very large. The problem with slaughtering in this way in facilities with large number of animals is cross contamination. Remember, I mentioned the E. coli infections that are toxic to humans. The E. coli becomes part of the cow's digestive tract when cows eat grains. Well, imagine having thousands of animals all with E. coli gut infections that are slaughtered in the same facility. The likelihood of contamination of the meat is very high. If bacteria like this E. coli gets released, you have a real problem. You may remember some of the E. coli outbreaks from the past. If not, you can read about them in the CNN article E-coli Outbreaks Fast Facts.[15].

Now remember, all of this could have been avoided, if the cattle had just been fed grass for the final days of their lives, as being fed grass for just 5 days eliminates the infection. This for some reason, which I will refrain from speculating about, is not being done. To counter this problem, large-scale slaughterhouses routinely wash their meat in some sort of antimicrobial agent.

Once the meat has been slaughtered and washed with toxic chemicals, it is sent to a processing house where other "things" are added to it. We already had hormones, antibiotics, and who knows what kind of anti-microbial wash, now they add more stuff to it? Yes, chemicals that promote shelf life, maintain color, and increased volume get added to the mix.

Exactly what is added is determined by the form of meat product being made? Some of the possibilities are:

CARI SCHAEFER, M.A., TCM, L.Ac.

- Salt (for taste, impact on meat proteins, shelf life)
- Nitrites (for curing color, flavor, shelf life)
- Ascorbic acid (to accelerate curing reaction)
- Phosphates (for protein structuring and water binding)
- Chemical preservatives (for shelf life)
- Antioxidants (flavor and shelf life)
- Monosodium glutamate MSG (enhancement of flavor)
- Food coloring substances (synthetic and of plant origin)[16]

Here are just a few examples of what these additives are known to do to your health.

According to the Mayo clinic, "It's thought that sodium nitrate may damage your blood vessels, making your arteries more likely to harden and narrow, leading to heart disease. Nitrates may also affect the way your body uses sugar, making you more likely to develop diabetes."[17]

In an article published in the U.S. National Library of Medicine titled *Phosphate Additive in Food – A Health Risk?*, the author stated, "It has recently been determined that phosphate additives in food may harm the health of persons with normal renal function. More recent studies have shown that the association between high phosphate concentrations and higher mortality is not restricted to persons with renal disease; it can also be observed in persons with cardiovascular disease and even in the general population."[18]

And if that is not enough, there is even more stuff added to meat in the form of fillers. These fillers mostly come from the grain and soy families. So if you have a food intolerance, like gluten, it is important that you learn all the ingredients in your meat. Turkeys are a perfect example. Do not assume your turkey is chemical and gluten free. Gluten is often injected into turkeys as part of a flavor enhancement strategy. Need I go on? There is more, but I think you get the point.

Where's the (Good) Beef?

To avoid eating animals that have been raised in these horrible conditions, to avoid the hormones, antibiotics, antimicrobial agents, and to avoid all the chemical additives, it is necessary to buy your meat raised in healthful ways. The problem is identifying who does that.

The USDA has no specific definition for "free-range" beef, pork, and other nonpoultry products. The best way to know if you are actually buying meat from an animal that was raised using those practices is to know your farmer. The best way to do this is, once again, shop at your local farmers market.

When you find a meat purveyor, ask how their meat is raised, where it is slaughtered, i.e., how far the animal must travel to the slaughterhouse, and how many animals are slaughtered at a time. If they are unable to answer these questions, then just move on. Most farmers who raise their animals in health-promoting ways are excited to talk about it.

You are looking for animals raised in a natural environment and processed close to home and in small numbers. If you find a grower you like, ask your local health food store to sell their products.

If you do not have a farmers market nearby, then search for a local CSA and see if they sell meat. If there are none, then search online. There are meat sellers who will ship their meat directly to you. I know I say local is best, but if local is not available, then having clean meat shipped to you is the next best option. Obviously, choose the closest supplier you can find. It is really not hard. It will just take some time. But the time is well worth it. You can even look up and contact the local chapter of the Westin Price foundation. They are dedicated to helping people find local healthy food sources.

One rancher I spoke to just the other day said, "Raising meat naturally is a labor of love." By buying meat from these kinds of ranchers, you are not only helping your health, you are also supporting the whole system of ranchers who want us to have good quality meat now and for the future to come.

FISH

Fish are a great protein source as well. They are also rich in fat-soluble vitamins, and omega 3s, an essential fatty acid for your health. They are good for our health in so many ways and yet...

Avoiding the C.R.A.P. Fish

The problem with fish is our oceans are becoming more and more polluted. Finding clean fish is becoming harder and harder. Now, not only do we have to be concerned about high mercury levels in fish like tuna but we also have to pay attention to high radiation levels due to the Fukishima nuclear accident.

I have found even one dose of tuna causing a problem for several clients. They come in, I test them, and mercury shows up. When I look at their food journal, they had recently eaten tuna.

Even though fish is a great source of protein and healthy fats, if it is fish loaded with toxins, and you may be doing yourself more harm than good.

I saw a bumper sticker once that summed it up "Friends do not let friends eat farm-raised fish." I had to chuckle. But it is true. Farm-raised fish are like CAFO raised cows. They are fed food that is not native to their diet, given antibiotics to counter infections, and raised in overcrowded conditions that promote infections and do not promote a healthy animal. When salmon are farm raised, due to alterations in their diet, they lose their pink color and are then dyed pink prior to selling.

As well, the first genetically modified animal likely to be approved for sale is salmon. At this writing, it is still being reviewed by the FDA, but it looks like they will vote in favor of it being allowed. In the near future, it is very likely that the farm-raised salmon you buy will be GMO.

Eating fish is a part of almost every healthy diet recommendation, but, as I said, how can eating a sick, toxic animal promote health? It just isn't logical. However, finding good sources is important, as healthy fish can play an important role in a healthy balanced diet.

Finding Food Forms of Fish Again

When you eat your fish, just make sure it is low in mercury, is not high in radiation, and wild caught. Avoid eating fish that live on the bottom such as catfish. Bottom-feeders tend to build up toxins in their tissue and, in most cases, eating shellfish is not a great idea for the same reason. You can do an Internet search to find out which local fish are the safest to eat.

Although shipping fish is not the most sustainable practice, if you do not live near a healthy fish source, it may be your only option for acquiring healthy animals. There is a company called Vital Choice that tests each catch for mercury levels and radiation levels. The fish is flash frozen on the boat, and it is some of the best tasting fish I have ever had. Plus they come in single serving packages that make using them very simple.

C.R.A.P. Meat & Fish	Food Form of Meat & Fish
✕ AFO-raised meat	✓ Meat raised in an animal-centered way
✕ CAFO-raised meat	✓ Free-range, grass-fed and finished meat
✕ Meat slaughtered in large slaughterhouse	✓ Free range, small-farm-raised chickens
✕ Meat sold in mass supermarkets	✓ Meat slaughtered at small slaughterhouses only
✕ Meat raised with antibiotics	✓ Locally raised meat as much as possible
✕ Meat fed on corn, soy, and other grains that are not part of their natural diet	✓ Healthy meat with fat intact
✕ Fish farm raised	✓ Wild-caught low-mercury and radiation fish
✕ Bottom-feeding fish	
✕ Fish high in mercury or radiation	

EGGS

Depending on your age, you may remember the campaign against eggs. Billboards all over the country were warning us against eating more than a few eggs a week. They were being blamed for causing elevated cholesterol. If you saw those billboards back then, you may have wondered why you no longer see them.

The reason is that there is nothing wrong with eggs. They will not raise your cholesterol. However, there is something wrong with unhealthy eggs from unhealthy chickens.

At the time that campaign was being promoted, the chickens in this country were being raised in such poor living conditions, fed all manner of unhealthful foods. The eggs they were producing were linked to health problems.

The growers cleaned-up their act and voila, suddenly eating eggs is not such a problem anymore.

This is a perfect example of how eating sick food will make you sick.

However, eggs in their natural healthy state are a great source of protein and healthy fat. And do not be fooled into thinking you should only eat the whites—the egg yolks are jam-packed full of important nutrients, especially the fat-soluble vitamins and they have more protein than the whites.

C.R.A.P. Eggs

How do you know you are eating healthy eggs? Unfortunately, reading the label is not the answer.

In the United States, the only free-range regulations that exist and are enforced by USDA are for poultry. Remember the regulation only indicates that the animal has been allowed access to the outside. It does not specify the quality or size of the outside range nor how much outside time an animal must have access to be considered free range.

In other words, the term "free range" doesn't really mean much. It is mostly used to get the consumer to pay more for the eggs, as are the terms "pasture-raised, "humanely raised," etc.

When I buy an egg from a "free-range" or "pasture-raised" chicken, I want an egg from an animal that gets to be outside in the sun and fresh air with room to hunt for worms and other bugs.

That brings up another point: any product that labels their eggs as "free range, vegetarian fed," is selling you a pile of marketing mumbo-jumbo.

Actually, what they are telling you is that you can be certain the egg is not from a free range or pasture-raised chickens. Chickens are not vegetarians by nature. They eat insects! So, if they are running around outside among plants, with bugs, it is impossible to keep them vegetarian.

Finding the Food Form of Eggs

The good news is it is pretty easy to tell if your eggs are fresh and healthy. When you crack an egg, the white should not spread out all over the pan. If it does then the egg is old. The yolk should be a rich orange color and should sit high up, instead of the flat anemic yolks most eggs provide. To find good quality fresh eggs, you have to find a local supplier. I was buying eggs from my local co-op from a farm that I really liked. I started recommending them to all my clients and then one day, I cracked open one of their eggs and it ran all over the pan and the yolk was a pale yellow and flat. Now, I had paid $7.50 for this carton of eggs, so I was not happy to be seeing that what I had just spent a lot of money buying was something I could have purchased at the local super market for a couple of bucks.

What often happens, and is the reason I do not recommend by brand, is that ethical growers get popular, are bought up by bigger growers, and gone are the practices that made the product good in the first place. Then, instead of buying the quality food you thought you were, you are only buying a familiar label. The food inside has nothing to do with the product you originally fell in love with.

So, once again, what's the best and easiest source of fresh eggs? You guessed it... your farmers market or other sources, like CSAs for local small egg producers. You might even consider getting a chicken or two of your own. Now that's fresh.

C.R.A.P. Eggs	Food Form of Eggs
✕ AFO-raised eggs	✓ Eggs from locally raised small farms purchased at the farmers market
✕ CAFO-raised eggs	✓ Eggs from pasture-raised chickens where they are free to eat bugs, etc.
✕ Eggs from caged chickens	✓ Eggs from chickens you and your family raise
✕ Labeled free-range eggs from the supermarket	
✕ Eggs from vegetable-fed chickens	

Fats and Oils

Nowhere have we been more mislead about food than about fats. In the late 1970s, it became very popular to demonize fat in this country, especially saturated fats. Fat was blamed for causing everything from high cholesterol to diabetes, plus heart disease and obesity.

It was and often still is presented as the evil cause of all our health problems. Low fat became the craze. Everything became low fat. The problem with low fat food, besides lacking essential naturally occurring nutrients, is that it is tasteless and leaves you wanting. To counter this, food manufacturers added in, you guessed it, sugar, and so, in my opinion, began the rapid downfall of American health.

Obesity has been linked to many, many health problems, and ever since low fat diets started being recommended, the obesity rates in this country have soared. So have diabetes, autoimmune disease, Alzheimer's, ADD, ADHD, depression, and anxiety.

Coincidence or direct cause? Good question. To answer this question, let's look at what I give to people that helps when they come into my clinic for all the above disorders. In every case, fat plays an important role.

Healthy fat is what helps a diabetic balance their blood sugar. Healthy fat is what helps obese people lose weight. Every autoimmune case I help requires healthy fats. Research has shown that Alzheimer's patients benefit from adding fat into the diet. And every ADD or ADHD case gets fats. The brain is made mostly of fat. How could low fat intake not play a role in a degenerating brain?

Why was fat demonized? It is my opinion that it was demonized because what we where eating were toxic fats. Hydrogenated oils, you know the stuff Crisco and margarine are made from, have been proven to raise cholesterol and promote heart disease and diabetes.

Also, remember toxins stick to fat, so when you are eating food loaded with pesticides, and other chemicals, the fat is going to be where those toxins settle. Eat the fat and you are eating the toxins.

If eating fat alone, especially saturated fat, were the cause of heart disease, then why would countries like Italy and France who have a diet much higher in saturated fats than ours have lower rates of heart disease than we do?

The United States ranks 29th in the world for incidence of diabetes while France is 101 and Italy is 129. How could fat be so unhealthy for us when countries that eat more fat, especially more saturated fat, are far healthier than we are here in the United States?

One thing that is known for certain is that since the recommendation was given to consumers in the United States to eat a lower fat diet, obesity rates have skyrocketed.

The Obesity Epidemic in the USA Started at Almost the Exact Same Time the Low-Fat Dietary Guidelines Were Published

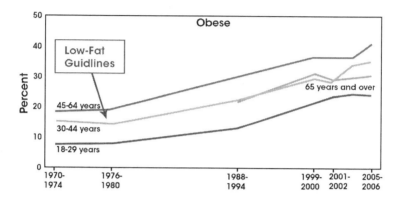

Source: National Center for Health Statistics (US). Health, United States, 2008: With Special Feature on the Health of Young Adults. Hyattsville (MD): National Center for Health Statistics (US); 2009 Mar. Chartbook.

So has the incidence of diabetes.

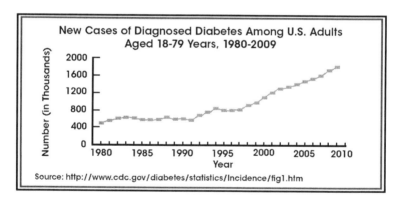

Limiting fat intake has certainly not solved some of the most common health problems here in this country. Has it contributed to the problem? Based on my clinical experience, I have to say yes.

I am willing to state unequivocally, based on years of clinical experience that eating healthy fat will not make you fatter, will not increase your risk of diabetes, and will not raise your cholesterol. It will, however, support healthy brain function, healthy balanced hormones, promote good skin quality, help your body heal, and promote an overall sense of well-being. But you do not have to believe me. All you have to do is stop eating toxic fats and add in healthy fats every day and see for yourself.

Finding the Good Fat

Make fat 20% to 35% of your daily calories. Fat has 9 calories a gram, so you have to eat fewer grams to meet your daily needs. Based on a 2,000-calorie-a-day diet, this amounts to about 400 to 700 calories a day, or about 44 to 78 grams of total fat. A tablespoon of coconut oil has 14 grams of fat. One cup of avocado has 21 grams. One ounce of macadamia nuts 22 grams, 4 ounces of dark meat without the skin 22 grams. A half-cup of whole milk mozzarella cheese 17 grams of fat. Getting enough fat in your diet is easy.

Also, make sure you are eating enough variety of fat, and not eating too many fats high in omega 6 and 9 verses omega 3. Do not worry too much about what that means if you're unfamiliar with this topic. It is enough to know that they are different nutrients found in fats. Know that omega 6 and 9 are found in avocado, olive oil, and sesame oil, and other vegetable oils and nuts. Omega 3s are found in fish such as salmon and sardines, raw dairy, pasture-raised eggs, meat from grass-fed, free-range animals, walnut oil, flax oil (must be converted in the body, not a great source for men as they do not convert the oil efficiently), and chia seeds, to name a few of the easiest obtainable sources of omega 3s.

Often, we are eating far more foods high in omega 6 and 9 than we are eating foods high in omega 3s. Too much omega 6 and not enough omega 3 increases inflammation in the system. Historically it was thought that humans ate a 1 to 1 ratio of omega 6 to omega 3. Today it is estimated that that ratio is more like 10 to 1 in some people, and can be as high as 25 to 1. Anything you do from a dietary perspective to bring that balance closer to the 1 to 1 ratio is going to help your health. Many alternative health practitioners savvy in diet say you can stretch the ratio to 3:1 or 4:1.

Eat only organic, cold-processed, and uncooked oils. When oil is cooked, it oxidizes. And oxidized oil is rancid. As soon as the oil is heated and mixed with oxygen, it goes rancid and should not be consumed. This is why I recommend avoiding cooked oils as much as possible.

Instead, learn to cook oil-free, adding oil to your food after it is cooked. You will be amazed at how simple it is to cook without oil. If it is necessary to cook with oil for a **special occasion,** then cooking with coconut oil for higher-temperature dishes such as baked goods, or butter and olive oil at low temperature are your best options as they are damaged less by heat than other oils.

All oil consumed must be cold-pressed, and organic. Flax oil is very volatile and should not be consumed unless freshness can be confirmed. Remember, flax oil should taste nutty and fresh. If it burns your throat, it is rancid and should be discarded, as it is toxic to your liver.

Coconut oil, other nut oils (except peanut oil), avocado, nuts and seeds, dark meat, and marbled meat from healthy animals, grass-fed organic butter, wild caught fish, and, raw dairy are all great sources of healthy fats.

Eat clean fats in moderation in a good balance of omega 6 to omega 3. It is a great thing you will do for your health.

C.R.A.P. Fats and oils	Food Form of Fats and Oils
✗ All processed oil	✓ Unprocessed, cold-pressed, organic oils
✗ All "vegetable oil"	✓ Coconut oil, walnut oil, olive oil, sesame seed oil, hazelnut oil, avocado oil all in glass only
✗ Corn oil	✓ Raw butter
✗ Canola oil	✓ Butter from pasture-raised cows
✗ Safflower oil	✓ Ghee from grass-fed cows
✗ Peanut oil	✓ Lard or fat from healthy, organic, pasture-raised, grass-fed animals
✗ Toasted sesame oil	✓ Fat and skin from healthy, organic, pasture-raised, grass-fed animals
✗ Rancid Flax oil	✓ Organic sprouted nuts & nut butters
✗ Crisco	✓ Organic pasture-raised eggs
✗ Margarine	✓ Raw whole-fat dairy products
✗ Butter from CAFO raised cows	✓ Raw cheese
✗ Grapeseed oil	
✗ Soy oil	
✗ Processed coconut oil	
✗ Olive oil that has been cut with other oils	
✗ Oil stored in plastic	

Salt

Since the dawn of civilization, salt has been used by humans to preserve and spice food. This being true, why in recent years, has salt, like fat, been demonized to the point where it is now considered a potential threat to our health? I made a conscious choice to avoid salt many years before my illness manifested, a choice I now know played a role in my health crisis.

The problem with eliminating salt is that salt is a required nutrient the body needs to survive. The reason it has been demonized has nothing to do with salt itself. The problem is similar to the fat problem; what matters most is the kind of salt we are eating. As with most of what is sold as food, salt has also been altered with added "stuff." It is these alterations, not the salt itself, that have taken it from being a health-supporting nutrient to a potential health hazard.

Having said that, sodium is sodium and no matter what form it is, it's still a necessary nutrient for the body. However, when you eat sodium in an isolated form devoid of other minerals that naturally occur, as is the case with table salt, you are creating imbalances in your system that, over time, can lead to health issues. Unfortunately, I found my health at the mercy of my choice to avoid table salt all together, and it wasn't pretty!

The ramification of this salt avoidance is rampant in my practice. After 15 years of working with clients, I find avoiding salt to be a recurring choice made by many who are chronically ill. "Oh no! I avoid salt at all cost!" I commonly hear.

Based on my experience, chronically sick people almost always have weak adrenals. Weak adrenals are often aggravated by salt avoidance, so the correlation between salt avoidance and poor adrenal health cannot be ignored.

Salt is the most abundant mineral used by the adrenal glands, two small glands that sit on top of the kidneys, to make adrenal hormones. They are small but critical not only for your well-being but also for your very survival, since they moderate your body's ability to adapt to stress.

A well-rounded diet of nutrient-dense food that includes salt is essential. Diet alone will not correct most cases of adrenal fatigue, but without dietary changes, adrenal health will not rebuild. Unfortunately, most adrenal-exhausted people I see do not eat well. Like I did, they often skip meals and eat limited diets that avoid salt, fat, and protein, all nutrients that play an essential role in adrenal health.

What's the moral of this story? Salt is essential, necessary, and mandatory, in fact, for the health of our adrenals. This begs the question: If it is so essential, why have we been told to avoid it? And how has it suddenly become this evil substance when man has been using it in food preparation since the very formation of civilization?

C.R.A.P. Salt

The reason for this is that we are not consuming salt in its natural form. The salt you buy at the grocery store and what passes for salt in most processed foods is made in a laboratory. It is highly processed to remove all trace elements until it is almost pure sodium and chloride. Once that part of the process is complete, other "things" are added to it such as Iodine and anti-caking agents.

Salt, when it comes from the earth or the sea, the way humans have consumed it for thousands of years, has a host of other intrinsic elements. These elements are known as trace minerals and are essential to our health.

Consuming iodized table salt in large quantities can deplete calcium, raise blood pressure, and promote hyperthyroidism and Hashimoto's thyroiditis. Eat processed food and you are consuming processed salt. And did I mention, it is added to everything? If you are consuming packaged processed foods, controlling your intake can be difficult. We need salt, just not the white stuff found on most tables in America.

Table salt, the kind you buy in the supermarket that is all white and pretty, is not a food. It is a chemical manufactured for appeal and shelf life and contains other substances and chemicals, added for just those reasons. Real salt is found in combination with other minerals and comes in many colors. Different trace minerals are different colors and tint the salt. Salt, in its natural form, will not be bright white.

Food Form of Salt

Now you may be thinking, can't I get enough salt from the food I eat? In theory, the answer should be yes. However, since mineral depletion in our soil, and hence our food, is a widespread problem, even eating a whole foods diet would benefit from adding a little extra natural salt.

I remember when I was first introduced to Himalayan salt. My practitioner told me to eat as much as I wanted. For about two weeks, I couldn't get enough. For those two weeks, I was a total salt fiend. Then I was done. There was something in it my body really needed and once that was satiated, the cravings stopped and my use became more moderate.

To find whole food salt, you can go to most health food stores. Some will sell it in bulk, which is a cost-effective way to purchase it. I like to vary my salt sources as well as the kinds of salt I use. By doing this, I increase the variety of minerals I am exposed to and decrease the potential exposure to any toxins that may be present in any one salt source.

Himalayan and Celtic Salt are two common names of whole food salt you may find on your health food store shelf. Try it. If you start to crave it, it is a good indicator that there is a mineral you are lacking that is in the salt. The cravings should balance out in a little while and then using salt in moderation is recommended. If however, your cravings do not subside, that could indicate an adrenal weakness that you may want to have evaluated by a qualified healthcare provider.

Before we leave the topic of salt and your health, let me say something about blood pressure. If you have high blood pressure, taking table salt, iodized white salt, out of your diet 100 percent, and I mean 100 percent, is a good idea. After you do, monitor your blood pressure for three weeks to see if you notice a change. If your blood pressure decreases, that is good to know, but even if it doesn't, keeping to a low table salt diet is a good choice.

Once you've eliminated table salt, don't stop there. Replace it with some salt from a natural source for a week. Monitor your blood pressure daily to see if you notice any changes that are consistent. Does the natural salt affect your blood pressure? In some cases, you may find your blood pressure lower with the natural salt. If adding in natural salt does not raise your blood pressure, then eliminating table salt from your diet and adding in some natural salt **in moderation** can be a health-promoting choice.

Every body is different. Pay attention to what your body, not your taste buds tell you about salt in your diet.

C.R.A.P. Salt	Food Form of Salt
✗ Iodized table salt	✓ Celtic sea salt
✗ Bleached salts	✓ Himalayan sea salt
	✓ Other whole salts (they will be a color other than white)

Water

By weight, your body is made up of more water than any other element. Water is an element that is in constant need of replenishing as a result of the normal everyday loss we experience through breath, perspiration, urine, and feces. For the body to function properly, we must be ever vigilant about replenishing our water supply on a daily basis.

Not only is water crucial for flushing toxins, it is also essential to carry nutrients to our organs, brain, and cells. It provides moisture for our nose, ears, throat, and skin providing a barrier that acts as a first line of defense for our immune system.

Lack of water can lead to dehydration, a condition that occurs when we don't have enough water and/or electrolytes (mineral salts such as sodium, calcium, chloride, magnesium and potassium) in our bloodstream to perform normal functions. Even mild dehydration can drain our energy and make us feel tired.

In today's reality, where toxic exposure is higher than ever, keeping our water consumption at optimum levels is even more critical. Without water, the body is unable to efficiently eliminate toxins, leaving our cells, organs, and tissues susceptible to damage.

Recommendations on the proper amount of water vary somewhat due to a number of variables. It's important to consider your body weight, how much exercise you get, how prone to perspiring you may be, or your susceptibility to losing excess water through loose or liquid bowels.

However, as a general rule, the range is 6 to 12 eight-ounce glasses of water per day, depending on your size. If you find it difficult to consume enough water, start with six glasses a day. If you are small, that may be enough. If you are taller or heavier, more is probably indicated.

If you tend to drink a lot of water, sticking to no more than 12 eight-ounce glasses is preferable. More than 12 is not necessary and is not necessarily better. Every time you eliminate water from the body through sweat, urine, or feces, you lose electrolytes. Electrolytes are essential to maintain life. They play a vital role in brain function and the proper function of your nervous system. If you are low in minerals to begin with, and then drink an excess of water without replacing minerals, you can actually become water toxic.

In severe cases, it is possible to develop a condition called hyperrhydration or water poisoning—a potentially fatal disturbance in brain function that results when the normal balance of electrolytes in the body becomes too low as a result of overconsumption of water.

Although water poisoning is an acute condition and only occurs under extreme conditions, less severe levels of water to electrolyte imbalance happen all the time. If you cannot satisfy your thirst no matter how much water you drink, you may be low in electrolytes. Drinking more water in this situation will only exacerbate your thirst as well as intensify the accompanying symptoms such as fatigue, low-grade headache, and heaviness in the limbs. The fatigue that usually accompanies a bout of diarrhea, vomiting, or a hangover is usually due to a loss of electrolytes.

Drinking more water without replenishing the nutrients can make the situation worse. Whenever I'm feeling extra thirsty or feel a need for a boost of electrolytes, I use this recipe.

- ½ tsp. Celtic or Himalayan sea salt
- ½ tsp. non-aluminum baking soda
- 1 quart water
- 125 ml orange juice, fresh is best
- ½ banana
- 1-½ tbs. raw honey

Blend and drink throughout the day. Remember, more water is not always better. Drink the proper amount for your body's needs and make sure you are getting your minerals through eating a balanced whole-food-based diet with plenty of leafy greens to maintain proper digestive function. Using Celtic sea salt and Himalayan sea salt will also help the body maintain proper electrolyte levels.

In the case of water, it is best to drink water that is slightly alkaline (7.5) with naturally occurring minerals. The way it is found in a natural spring.

When water is consumed that has a much higher pH, such as the case with the current alkaline water craze in California, where people are being encouraged to drink water with a pH of 8.5 or 9, health issues arise.

In my opinion, based on the clients I have seen, drinking high alkaline water will, in the end actually lead to mineral deficiencies in the body and the excess unabsorbed minerals can accumulate in the kidneys and cause kidney stones.

If you want to maintain a good pH, make sure your digestive tract is functioning optimally, eat lots of vegetables and kelp (not from Japan), both rich in minerals, and avoid foods that are lacking in minerals like processed flours, breads, pasta, processed sugars, and, in general, any processed food at all.

Drinking purified water is a must, since our tap water is loaded with so many chemicals that it cannot be considered safe for consumption. That said, I do not recommend water in plastic bottles either, as it has been found in several different studies with various types of plastics that they are leaching harmful chemicals into the water.[19]

To solve this issue, I only recommend drinking filtered water, or water that is delivered to you in glass.

As of this writing, August 2015, a few companies will deliver water to your home in glass bottles. Or you can purchase an in-home filtration system. There are many varieties. You will need to do a little research about the best sources for your water. Unfortunately, things change so quickly that if I recommended one here, it may no longer be available in your area by the time you read this. Currently, I use a combination of a counter-top Berkey System with extra fluoride filters and Mountain Valley Spring Water delivered in glass.

C.R.A.P. Water	Food Form of Water
✗ Water from the tap	✔ Water that has been filtered to remove chlorine, chloramines, heavy metals, micro-organisms, and fluoride
✗ Water that has been stored in plastic	✔ Water stored in glass
✗ Water that has had the pH altered to be above 7.5	✔ Water with a pH of 7.5
✗ Water that is softened	

Sugar: Looking for the Sweet Life

What would a book on food be without talking about sugar, and how can we talk about sugar without talking about sugar cravings?

Sugar is a naturally occurring substance in food. You cannot avoid it. Neither do you want to— sugar in the form of glucose is very important to your body. It is a main ingredient your body uses to make energy. It is essential. That said, sugar has become a very big problem and it is now contributing to numerous health problems.

Note: Actually, we can live without sugar! Humans can live without carbohydrates and do so for several months, as what has occurred in survival situations.

Here in the United States, we are obsessed with adding sugar to everything. You can find added sugar in dairy products, pasta sauces, bread products, and even meat. We add it to so many foods that the USDA estimates the average person consumes 156 pounds per year of added sugar! That is 31 five-pound bags for each of us.[20]

That is a staggering number, especially when you understand the devastating effects too much sugar can have on your body.

Our body has several ways to combat low blood sugar, a condition that arises when food is not consumed for several hours and blood glucose levels drop too low to supply the body's needs. There is, however, only one system designed to protect you from high blood sugar.

We are not designed to overeat sugar. When processed and / or added sugar enters the body, it moves into the bloodstream very rapidly leading to a blood glucose surge. Every time you eat something with added sugar, you are placing a stress on your body that it has to respond to. And that response is to convert the excess sugar to fat.

Not only are you promoting the production of fat and, hence, weight gain, when cells are bombarded with too much sugar too often, they close their doors. The cells become resistant to the hormone that moves sugar into the cell, and Type II diabetes can set in. Once diabetes sets in, you are at a greater risk for several serious health problems.

Because sugar molecules are large, when there are too many of them in your blood, you run the risk of damaging small capillaries found in places like your feet, organs such as your kidneys, or your eyes. Wounds become slow to heal due to poor blood flow. This is why people who have diabetes run an increased risk for foot amputations, blindness, and/or developing kidney failure as happened with my father.

Some of the latest research on Alzheimer's is finding a diabetes-like environment in the brain as the source of cell destruction. Much like in diabetes, brain cells lose their ability to move glucose across the cell wall. Without glucose, they are unable to make energy, without energy they die, leading to the devastating brain deterioration found in Alzheimer's patients.[21]

These are just a few of the health problems arising at alarming rates in this country from the overconsumption of sugar, and this is just the beginning.

Immune challenges such as pathogenic bacteria, fungi, and parasites, as well as cancer cells all make energy through a process called fermentation. Sugar is used to fuel this process. When blood glucose levels are high, you are providing a great environment for immune challenges and cancer cells to thrive. Is high sugar consumption, a reason for the increase in cancer rates? In my opinion, it is a possibility that should not be ignored, especially if you already have cancer.

So, if sugar is so bad, then why do we crave it so much? Why is sugar such a temptation for many of us, often one of the most difficult habits to shift?

That is a really good question. It is a good question because sugar cravings are often the first sign of a developing health problem, and are often your body's attempt at solving a problem.

If your blood sugar drops too low, as can happen when you chronically skip meals or eat a high-sugar meal without protein and fat, or have weakened adrenal glands, you will crave sugar. It will literally be impossible to walk by that piece of candy or sticky bun. At the point that the blood sugar is low enough, your brain will do anything to increase supplies and the quickest way to do that is a simple sugar source such as white flour, or candy. When it comes to blood sugar lows, your will power will lose every time.

Sugar also has the effect of giving you a short-term boost in serotonin, the neurotransmitter responsible for feeling happy. So, again, you may not be suffering from weak willpower, you may be unknowingly trying to treat depression. Women, did you ever wonder why you crave sugar before your cycle. You guessed it, that little mood boost. It just takes the edge off. The problem is, it only takes the edge off for a moment and then you end up lower than when you started.

Sugar, as I mentioned, supports immune challenges to thrive. In my clinic, it is common to find an overload of some sort of bug, such as a bacteria or fungus, when a person is suffering from sugar cravings. Once the bug is under control, the sugar cravings just melt away like magic.

If you are craving sugar after meals, you may be in the beginning stages of diabetes. Sugar cravings before meals with an increased sensitivity to sugar consumption might be pointing towards adrenal fatigue affecting your system.

If you are having sugar cravings, then you may be heading down the road to a more serious health problem. Seeking support around identifying why you are having the cravings is very important.

Not all sugar sources have the same effect on the body. Obviously, sugar that is naturally occurring in food is going to have a less negative affect than added sugar. However, the problem is that once you have an immune challenge, such as a fungal infection, weakened adrenals, or a condition like pre-diabetes, often, even naturally occurring sugar in foods such as fruit can aggravate that health challenge, making a very restrictive diet necessary until the problem is under control.

Why wait until it is medically necessary to decrease your sugar intake?

If, during The 21-Day Diet Detox, you crave sugar, see if it helps to drink some water and/or eat half an avocado. Sometimes, your craving is really a need for water or healthy fat.

But if you try these things and, by the end of the detox, you are still dealing with sugar cravings, then I suggest you seek the support of a medical professional. You may have to find someone who practices preventative medicine. They should be able to help you identify what is behind your sugar cravings.

A Few C.R.A.P. Forms of Sugar Worth an Added Note

White sugar is a negative food. All substances require nutrients to process. When you eat a food like white sugar and white flour, you are consuming only glucose without any of the cofactors necessary to process the sugar, so your body has to take from its own stores. In doing so, minerals are leached from your body, making you less nutrient-dense after eating than you were before. Eating negative foods defeats the most important purpose for why we eat.

From a health perspective, high fructose corn syrup is a nightmare. It has been linked to an increase in diabetes and obesity. I would never let children eat it and I certainly wouldn't eat it myself. I know it means no Heinz ketchup, but trust me; the short-term pleasure just isn't worth the potential health challenge.

Artificial sweeteners in diet food and drinks are just as bad! They are chemicals, not food, and they all come with some form of a negative side effect. When fed to lab animals, they have been found to do such horrible things like deteriorate brain cells, promote cancer growth, and, believe it or not, promote weight gain.

It is a far better strategy to balance your sugar cravings than try to use potentially dangerous chemicals to nullify them.

Alcohol sugars are any chemicals that end in 'ol' on the label. They give you diarrhea if eaten in too large a quantity. I learned this the hard way some years ago as I sat on the freeway in dead stop traffic, eating a bag of sugar free candy. I came very close to having an accident, and I do not mean with another car. The body gets diarrhea when it is trying to eliminate something that is either toxic or irritating to the system.

Splenda is basically chlorine mixed with white sugar.

Stevia, on the other hand, is an herb that can actually help balance blood sugar. The problem is the stevia you are most likely buying has been processed and had other "things" added to it, making it a processed food instead of an herb. Stevia comes from a plant and, in its natural form, is green. If you are **not** consuming a green powder or pure stevia liquid, then what you are ingesting is no longer stevia in its food form.

Food Form of Sugar

Eat as little added sugar as possible. Try eating foods like sweet potatoes and yams. They are sweet in flavor and will nourish your body rather than just give you the temporary sweet fix. If you feel like having dessert then research where you can find, or how you can make raw desserts. Unlike standard desserts that are loaded with added sugar and often contain processed flours, raw desserts are made fresh, contain sweeteners that come from natural sources like raw honey or dates and are loaded with good fats and other nutrients.

Following The 21-Day Diet Detox is the first step to eliminating sugar cravings. Often, after the 3 weeks, you will be amazed at how little you crave it.

C.R.A.P. Sugar	Food Form of Sugar
✕ White & brown sugar	✓ Sugar naturally occurring in food.
✕ Alcohol sugars; anything on a label with (ol) at the end (sorbitol, mannitol, xylitol, etc.)	✓ Dates, and other fruit
✕ Artificial sugar substitutes; Sweet & Low (saccharine) sucrose, Equal & Nutrasweet (aspartame), Splenda, Truvia (processed stevia)	✓ Green leaf stevia
✕ High fructose corn syrup	✓ Raw honey
✕ Fructose	✓ Raw desserts
✕ Dextrose	✓ In limited amounts; molasses, cane sugar, raw agave, coconut sugar, and lou han guo
✕ Non-raw agave	

END NOTES

1. Torsten Bohn, Lena Davidsson, Thomas Walczyk, and Richard F Hurrell, "Phytic acid added to white-wheat bread inhibits fractional apparent magnesium absorption in humans," *American Journal of Clinical Nutrition* 79, no. 3 (March 2004): 418-423, accessed September 1, 2015, http://ajcn.nutrition.org/content/79/3/418. abstract#aff-1

2. B. Lönnerdal, A. S. Sandberg, and C. Kunz, "Inhibitory effects of phytic acid and other inositol phosphates on zinc and calcium absorption in suckling rats," Journal of Nutrition 119, no. 2 (1989): 211-214, accessed September, 2015, http://jn.nutrition.org/content/119/2/211.full.pdf

3. "Chapter 2: Profiling Food Consumption in America" In Agricultural Fact Book, accessed August 28, 2015, http://www.usda.gov/factbook/chapter2.pdf

4. Laura Newcomer, "What's Up With Modern Wheat?http://greatist.com/health/modern-wheat-health-gluten," December 10, 2012, accessed August 28, 2015.

5. "The Bread and Flour Regulations 1998 (as amended): Guidance Notes," accessed August 28, 2015,http://www.food.gov.uk/sites/default/files/multimedia/pdfs/breadflourguide.pdf

6. Joseph M. Mercola, "The Little-Known Secrets about Bleached Flour," March 26, 2009, accessed August 28, 2015, http://articles.mercola.com/sites/articles/archive/2009/03/26/The-Little-Known-Secrets-about-Bleached-Flour.aspx

7. Banu. M, Shakila and P. Sasikala, "Alloxan in refined flour: A Diabetic concern," International Journal of Advanced and Innovative research, no. 2278-7844 (2012): 204-209, accessed August 28, 2015, http://ijair.jctjournals.com/sept2012/t12930.pdf

8. "Where did all the baby boys go?" New Scientist (August 31, 2005), accessed August 28, 2015, http://www.newscientist.com/article/mg18725154.800

9. Paul B. Kaplowitz and Sharon E. Oberfield, "Reexamination of the Age Limit for Defining When Puberty Is Precocious in Girls in the United States: Implications for Evaluation and Treatment," Pediatrics 104, no. 4, (October 1, 1999): 936, accessed August 28, 2015, http://pediatrics.aappublications.org/content/104/4/936.short

10. "What are amino acids?" last modified July, 2015, accessed August 28, 2015, http://www.aminoacid-studies.com/amino-acids/what-are-amino-acids.html

11. H. Roger Segelken, "Simple change in cattle diets could cut E. coli infection,"
Cornell Chronical (Sept. 8, 1998), accessed August 28, 2015, http://www.news.cornell.edu/stories/1998/09/simple-change-cattle-diets-could-cut-e-coli-infection

12. EPA, "What is a CAFO?" accessed August 28, 2015, http://www.epa. gov/region7/water/cafo/

13. Matthew Hoffman, "Safer Food For a Healthier You," December 18, 2008, accessed August 28, 2015, http://www.webmd.com/diet/ features/safer-food-healthier-you

14. M. E. Lippman, K. A. Krueger, S. Eckert, A. Sashegyi, E. L. Walls, S. Jamal, J. A. Cauley, and S. R. Cummings, "Indicators of lifetime estrogen exposure: effect on breast cancer incidence and interaction with raloxifene therapy in the multiple outcomes of raloxifene evaluation study participants," Journal of Clinical Oncology 19, no. 12(2001 Jun 15, 2001): 3111-3116, accessed August 28, 2015, http:// www.ncbi.nlm.nih.gov/pubmed/11408508

15. "E-Coli Outbreaks Fast Facts," last modified June 10, 2015, accessed August 28, 2015http://www.cnn.com/2013/06/28/ health/e-coli-outbreaks-fast-facts

16. "Non-Meat Ingredients," accessed August 28, 2015, http://www.fao. org/docrep/010/ai407e/AI407E06.htm

17. Katherine Zeratsky, "Does the Sodium Nitrate in Processed Meat Increase My Risk of Heart Disease?" April 10, 2015, accessed August 15, 2015, http://www.mayoclinic.org/healthy-living/nutrition-and-healthy-eating/ expert-answers/sodium-nitrate/faq-20057848

18. Eberhard Ritz, Kai Hahn, Markus Ketteler, Martin K Kuhlmann, and Johannes Mann, "Phosphate Additives in Food—a Health Risk," Deutsches Arteblatt International 109, no. 4 (January 27, 2012): 49–55, accessed August 28, 2015, http://www.ncbi.nlm.nih.gov/pmc/ articles/PMC3278747/

19. Chun Z. Yang, Stuart I. Yaniger, V. Craig Jordan, Daniel J. Klein, George D. Bittner, "Most Plastic Products Release Estrogenic Chemicals: A Potential Health Problem That Can Be Solved," *Environmental Health Perspective* 119, no.7 (July 2011): 989-996, accessed September 1, 2015, http://jn.nutrition.org/content/119/2/211.full.pdf

20. Jon Casey, "The Hidden Ingredient That Can Sabotage Your Diet," accessed August 29, 2015, http://www.medicinenet.com/script/main/ art.asp?articlekey=56589

21. F. G. De Felice, M. V. Lourenco, and S. T. Ferreira, "How Does Brain Insulin Resistance Develop in Alzheimer's Disease?" *Alzheimer's and Dementia* 10, no. 1 Suppl(February, 2014): S26-32, accessed on August 29, 2015, http://www.ncbi.nlm.nih.gov/pubmed/24529521

CHAPTER 7

Designing The Diet
That Is Right For You

The right "diet" or way for you to eat is the one that you like that meets the needs of your body. I know you may be thinking, "But I like pasta and white bread and cupcakes." However, that diet is not going to support you in your goal of good health. So, a better statement would be…the diet that is right for you is the diet that supports you in achieving the health you want and that you enjoy.

In designing this diet, you must be willing to try new things, branch out, and educate yourself a bit. If I gave you a diet plan to follow, you would most likely do what millions of other people have done when they tried the latest fad diet, do it for a while and then stop.

Instead, follow these guidelines, regardless of the diet you choose, and you will be doing a lot to make sure you are giving your body what it needs to be healthy.

The following guidelines will assure that you are eating a diet that is rich in nutrients, free of chemicals, and is supplying you with what your body needs to stay healthy.

1. Variety is the key.
2. Eat it whole and eat it fresh.
3. Make sure your diet includes enough protein.

4. Keep your blood sugar balanced: It is essential for your long-term health.
5. Make friends with vegetables.
6. Eat a combination of cooked and raw food.
7. Eat just enough and avoid overeating.
8. Change where you shop.
9. Change where and how often you eat out.
10. Travel wisely; travel prepared…Secrets to traveling and eating healthy.
11. Everything in moderation is okay.

Guideline #1: Variety is the Key!

We are meant to eat a variety of foods. This is because foods contain different nutrients, and if we eat the same foods over and over, we will be creating an imbalance in the nutrients the body is getting. It's also because foods can contain substances that can have a negative effect on the body. If we are always eating the same thing, we may be inadvertently predisposing ourselves to a health problem.

Here's a story about one of my clients named Mary. Mary lived far away so we really needed our sessions to be as impactful as possible, as driving back and forth required hours of her time and aggravated her arthritis pain, her chief complaint.

New clients always bring in a 3-day record of what they have been eating. When I asked to see hers, she was very eager to share. She was even a little proud of it.

I looked it over and I had to admit it looked pretty good. She was eating all organic. "I love to shop at the farmers market," she exclaimed. She was eating in a way that balanced her blood sugar, and she was cooking mostly at home.

Great! Diet is such an important part of arthritis management, and having that piece already handled would make my job a lot easier. However, when I looked a little closer, I noticed that almost every day for lunch she had stew. When I asked about it, she smiled boldly. "Oh, I love that stew. I make it all the time; it's my favorite."

I asked her what the ingredients were, and she told me it included some form of meat, potatoes, tomatoes, eggplant, red, and yellow bell peppers, some onion and zucchini, as well as oregano, sage, parsley and cayenne pepper for flavor.

As I was listening, my heart began to sink. "Sounds delicious," I said, wanting to encourage her great efforts to cook for herself. "And yet, there is one problem; almost everything in that stew increases pain. They are all what we call nightshades."

Her face dropped. I went on to explain how when people are in pain, it is recommended that they avoid nightshades as much as possible. She unknowingly was eating a pain stew every day.

Supporting someone with arthritis takes time. By changing the ingredients of her stew and avoiding the nightshades, her pain level reduced significantly.

Situations like this happen more often than not. Remember, it is usually the choices we make every day that affect our health. Eating a variety of foods will assist you in not making the mistake Mary made. If you eat a variety of foods, then you do not need to worry yourself with whether you are unknowingly creating a problem.

Different colored vegetables have different nutrients. Eat a wide range of colors and you are eating a wide range of nutrients. Different meats have different effects on the body—eat a variety and you will be getting a variety of nutrients. The same is true for grains and legumes.

Different foods have different effects on the acid levels of the body. Vegetables are more alkaline; meats and grains are more acidic. Balance your intake and you will be naturally eating a diet that balances your body's pH. If you adopt a diet that excludes certain food groups like a vegetarian or vegan diet, which can be very alkaline, then learn about foods that are acidic that fit within your dietary parameters. Remember, the blood is maintained at a pH of 7.2, slightly alkaline. If you eat a diet that is too alkaline, you can actually create imbalances due to too much alkalinity.

Following are some charts of the foods that contain nutrients that can pose a problem if eaten in too large a quantity. You do not need to go crazy memorizing these lists, or worrying about them.

Just look them over and make sure you are not eating, or adding in a lot of foods from one group.

Oxalic acid containing foods, can predispose the body to develop kidney stones, and can play a role in bladder irritation and inflammation.

Foods high in oxalic acid include:

Foods high in oxalic acid include:		
Beets	Ground pepper	Rhubarb
Soy	Lamb	Sorrel
Beet tops	Lime peel	Spinach
Black tea	Nuts	Swiss chard
Chocolate	Parsley	
Figs	Poppy seeds	

Goitrogenic foods, when eaten often in high amounts and in their raw form, can suppress the function of the thyroid. They include:

Goitrogenic foods		
Cassava, when crushed and unsoaked	Spinach	Chinese cabbage
Soybeans edamame (and soybean byroducts; tofu, soybean oil, soy flour, Hyphenate soy based protein powders)	Sweet potatoes	Collard greens
Pine nuts	Bok choy	Horseradish
Peanuts	Broccoli	Kale
Flax seeds	Broccolini	Kohlrabi
Millet	Brussels sprouts	Mustard greens
Strawberries	Cabbage	Radishes
Pears	Canola	Rutabagas
Peaches	Cauliflower	Turnips

Nightshades can aggravate pain and inflammation:

Nightshades	
Bell peppers (sweet peppers)	Paprika
Eggplant	Potatoes (but not sweet potatoes)
Goji berries (a.k.a. wolfberry)	Tomatillos
Pimentos	Tomatoes
Hot peppers (chili peppers, jalapenos, habaneros, chili-based spices, red pepper, cayenne)	

Guideline #2: Eat it whole and eat it fresh.

Often, when I talk about eating a whole-food diet, people stare at me blankly. I see the glaze going over their eyes. Once in a while, a brave soul will exclaim, "Excuse me, but what the heck does eating a whole-food diet mean exactly? I hear people talk about it all the time, but I have no idea what that means."

Do not despair; if you feel the same way, you are not alone. Let's make it as simple as possible.

Eating a whole-food diet means eating foods as close to their natural state as possible. Eating foods that have little to no added chemicals have not been ground and then stored on a shelf prior to eating. For example, if you are eating rice, have brown rice instead of rice pasta for a more whole-food choice. If you are eating a cereal for breakfast, putting cooked grains in the blender and adding your favorite milk choice is a more whole-food option than buying a boxed creamed cereal.

Eating foods in the natural state does have a caveat. As you have read in the previous chapters, some foods in their natural state have things in them that actually hinder digestion. This is where the art of food preparation comes in.

One mistake I see being made in the American diet is we are so obsessed with fast everything, that a large portion of what we eat has been ground-up in one form or another days, weeks, and, sometimes, even months before we consume it. This includes everything from our flour-laden diets to our protein powder craze.

Once food has been ground up, the nutrients that were otherwise protected in an outer wall are now exposed to oxygen, and oxygen changes things. It alters minerals, oxidizes fats, and degrades vitamins.

Orange juice that has been freshly squeezed loses a majority of its vitamin C in just minutes. Why do you think they fortify the orange juice you buy in the grocery store with vitamin C?

Flax seeds are another great example. Flax oil is a very unstable oil. Instability in an oil means it goes rancid very easily. Although, flax oil can have some good health benefits, if it is eaten rancid, it is very toxic to the liver. If your flax oil does not taste nutty and fresh or if it burns your throat or tastes bitter, then throw it away.

When I first learned this about flax, every time a client would bring in their flax oil in gel caps, I would crack one open and taste the oil. The oil was rancid every time. After doing this about a half dozen times, having bitter foul tasting oil in my mouth, I learned my lesson. Now, if my clients want to know if their flax oil is fresh, they have to do their own taste test. Because the oils in flax are so sensitive to oxygen, flax seed should be eaten only if consumed within hours of being ground. Throw away any of your containers of ground flax at home.

The oils in flour go rancid within three days of being ground. If you happen to find a whole-grain bread that has been fermented prior to baking, as is needed to enhance digestibility, good luck on finding one that is less than three days old. You are eating a bunch of rancid oils, which is a real health problem in and of itself.

In a perfect world, we would be able to buy bread that was made from freshly ground flour that has been fermented prior to baking. It really is not a lot to ask for. It is how bread has been made for thousands of years. The problem is that, in this country, it seems to be next to impossible to find.

No, I am not saying never eat bread, that would be unrealistic for most people, but do not be fooled into thinking that bread, pasta, cereal, or even your instant oatmeal are nutritious. They are not. Instead, use them as placeholders, and count them as a good dose of glucose, and then ask yourself, "Now where am I going to get my nutrition?"

This is a good rule to follow with any meal that includes products made from flours. Think of it as food for your soul rather than food for your body.

For example, have pasta. Instead of a lot of pasta with a little red sauce and a little cheese, have a little pasta with a lot of nutrient-dense vegetables.

Instead of that nutrition bar that is all ground up, choose one that has the nuts in larger pieces. Or forget the bar altogether and eat some sprouted nuts and a few dates, it is the same thing after all, just in a different shape with a lot more nutrition for less money.

Guideline #3: Make sure your diet includes enough protein.

Protein is essential for life to exist. Remember, enzymes are made from the amino acids that come from protein. They are required to make all chemical reactions happen in the body. For humans to be alive, chemical reactions must be occurring all the time, so protein is essential for life to continue. Some amino acids the body can make; others you must consume.

Rather than making yourself crazy with worrying about it, make sure you are varying your sources of protein.

Protein from animal sources is more easily digested and, therefore, available to the body; however, you can get your protein from a plant-based diet. If you choose to eat a low-meat, or mostly plant-based diet, you must make sure you educate yourself about where you are getting protein from and if you are getting enough. One of the common dietary mistakes I see in my clinic is women not eating enough protein to meet their body's needs.

General recommendations of protein needs vary. Here is an easy way to estimate your protein needs.

If you are active, or when your body is stressed and healing, the demand for protein goes up. Based on your activity level, take your body weight and multiply it by the number below and you will get an estimate of the amount of protein in grams that is right for your body.

Sedentary	Weight in pounds X .4
Active	Weight in pounds X .6
Competitive athlete	Weight in pounds X .75
Light body-builder	Weight in pounds X .85

If you are under a lot of stress and/or healing and not very active, multiply your body weight times .6 to estimate your body's needs. However, in doing this, decrease the amount of starchy foods you eat, so you do not gain weight from overeating.

How to estimate protein in food:

- A 3-ounce piece of meat has approximately 21 grams of protein (about the average sized person's palm)
- A 3-ounce piece of fish about 16 grams
- One egg has 6 grams of protein

Beans or legumes, nuts, and grains vary, depending on the grain, and amounts can be easily found with a quick Internet search, on the label, if you are buying your grains and legumes packaged in bags, or on the bin label if you are buying them in bulk.

For example, 1 cup of almonds has 30 grams of protein. However, unlike meat and egg protein, beans, nuts, and grains are not complete proteins, so different kinds of foods must be combined together in a day to make sure you are eating all the essential amino acids. A grain with a legume or bean, for example, has all the essential amino acids.

If you choose to eat a low to no meat diet, taking some time to research where you will get your complete protein will help to keep you healthy. Hemp seeds, buckwheat, and quinoa are some of the few plants sources of complete proteins. Beyond that, it becomes necessary to combine your foods together to obtain a complete amino-acid profile. Doing a little research to learn what foods make good combinations to assure you are eating all the amino acids you require is a great idea![1]

A note about protein powders as a solution

In my clinical experience, protein powders can be used for a short-term cleanse, or to fill in a need when we travel or some other factor limits our protein intake. However, because protein powders have been altered from their original form, isolated from their cofactors, and ground into a powder, they are not a whole food. I have not seen a protein powder that was able to support the body in the same way as eating food does. If you need one, then use it for a short period of time, make sure it is made from food (except soy) and not in a lab, and return to eating food as soon as possible.

Guideline #4: Keep your blood sugar balanced: It is essential for your long-term health.

The biggest mistake I see clients make is eating erratically. Every time your blood sugar goes too high, your body stores fat. However, every time your blood sugar is too low your body goes into a stress response. One of the major sources of internal stress I see is unbalanced blood sugar. Now, most of you have heard that when you eat too much sugar, you are putting yourself at risk for developing type 2-diabetes, but when your blood sugar is chronically dropping too low, you are also putting yourself at risk of developing health challenges.

One of the very frequent health challenges I see in my practice in Los Angeles is exhausted adrenals. It is the job of the adrenals to regulate blood sugar. If your blood sugar drops too low, your adrenals release cortisol to signal the liver to break down stored sugar. However, cortisol does a whole lot of other things. When cortisol is released, the body does not pick and choose what effects it will have, so a stress response is triggered. You can do everything "right" from a diet perspective, but if you skip enough meals or eat the wrong food combinations, you may find yourself feeling really stressed out. If this goes on long enough, then you can end up with exhausted adrenals.

If you are waking up in the night, but are able to fall back asleep, you may be in the first stages of adrenal weakness. If you find yourself wide-awake in the night, unable to fall back asleep, chances are your adrenals are pretty wiped out.

Stacy came into my practice complaining that she woke up every day feeling shaky and anxious. We ran a comprehensive blood test and an adrenal panel on her and found that her adrenals were so weak that they were no longer able to balance her blood sugar.

When this happens, the body is unable to regulate blood sugar through the night. When blood sugar levels drop too low, the adrenals release cortisol and you wake up. Or in an even more dramatic experience, if cortisol levels are too low and thereby not available, then the body will use adrenalin. When this happens, you wake up in a full-blown stress response before your foot even hits the floor, as was the case with Stacy.

If you have ever woken in the middle of the night with fear for no reason, then you have probably experienced a middle-of-the-night adrenaline surge. If you are waking up and unable to eat, lacking in appetite, then your body has probably already corrected your low blood sugar, and you are now in a stress response. Remember, cortisol suppresses appetite. Add some coffee to the mix and you are rearing to start the day. The only problem is that your body is running on borrowed fuel with nothing to back it up. In other words, you are running on fumes. Do this long enough and you can literally lose your ability to do anything at all, as in the case of chronic fatigue.

If you are experiencing any of these scenarios, then you most likely have some level of adrenal fatigue and would be very wise to regulate your blood sugar.

Repairing basic blood sugar regulation guidelines are as follows:

- Wait no more than 14 hours between dinner and your next meal.
- Eat 3 meals a day consisting of about 21 grams of protein (a 3-ounce piece of meat for example), 27 grams of carbohydrates (examples are ½ cup rice or 6 cups of kale) and a tablespoon of healthy oil or a small amount of a fatty food like an avocado or nuts.
- 2 ½ hours after a meal, have a snack consisting of 1 ounce of animal protein, or 7 grams of plant based protein and 7 grams of carbs, plus a teaspoon of fat.
- If, after an hour, you don't have time to eat your next meal, have another snack, repeat until you are able to have another meal.
- Before bed, have a snack in the amount suggested above.
- If you are overweight, make sure you stay within the limits listed above. If you are underweight, you can increase your quantity—just stay within the ratios stated. In most cases, regulating blood sugar will not fix adrenal fatigue alone;

however, without regulating your blood sugar, you will not fix your adrenal fatigue.

When I first learned about this, I was surprised to discover I was eating too much protein and not enough carbohydrates to balance my blood sugar. Paying attention to how you are eating and in what balance for a period of time can help you learn how to naturally make food choices that are balanced without much thought. Once you apply the effort to learn the basics, then it can become a natural way of life.

Guidelines #5: Make friends with vegetables.

Vegetables should be the majority of our food intake. Vegetables are rich in minerals, vitamins, amino acids, fiber, and other phytonutrients necessary for a human body to sustain life optimally.

For optimal health, it is best to choose to eat a ratio of not less than ¾ vegetables to ¼ fruit. The fruit available today has been hybridized to be much sweeter, i.e., contain more sugar, than fruit of the past.

On the list below, circle vegetables you enjoy eating, are willing to eat, and those you haven't tried, but are willing to. Cross out the ones you "know" for sure are a no.

Each week, try adding a new vegetable to a meal, making note of the ones you like. Remember, variety is the key.

Organic Vegetables to Try

Artichoke
Asparagus
Acorn Squash
Beets
Bok Choy
Broccoli
Broccoflower
Broccolini
Butternut squash

Brussels sprouts
Cabbage
Carrots
Cauliflower
Celery
Celery Root
Chard
Cilantro
Cucumber

Eggplant	Pumpkin
Kale	Radish
Kohlrabi	Rhubarb
Leafy Green (any)	Rutabaga
Leek	Shallots
Lettuce-any (except ice-burg)	Spinach
Mustard Greens	Spaghetti Squash
Okra	Sweet Potato
Onions	Tomatoes
Parsnip	Turnips
Parsley	Watercress
Peas	Yams
Peppers (green, red, orange,	Yellow Squash
yellow)	Zucchini

Guideline #6: Eat a combination of cooked and raw food.

There is a long-standing debate as to whether cooking vegetables or consuming them raw is best. The "raw" argument posits that when food is cooked, enzymes found in the food needed to digest it are destroyed, and water-soluble vitamins are destroyed.

Advocates of cooked food, upon which my background in Chinese medicine is based, argue that eating raw is very weakening to the digestive system and can lead to health challenges.

So which is true? Actually, they both are. When cooking food, certain nutrients and enzymes will be damaged and/or destroyed. However, when eating only raw, you can also lose the benefit of phytonutrients that are locked in the fiber of the food. Once cooked, those nutrients are unbound and available to your body.

Our digestive enzymes are very sensitive to temperature. Therefore, if you are eating a diet of raw, cold food, you may inadvertently be hindering their functions. However, the enzymes that naturally occur in food will be altered from cooking.

A diet of moderation, which includes both cooked and raw, will create balance in the body. Royal Lee has been quoted as saying that no more than 50% cooked vegetables is best. If you live in a cold climate, eat more cooked foods in the winter and more raw foods in the warmer months, but eat both cooked and raw. This way, you will not be losing out on any of the nutrients.

Moderation, Moderation, Moderation! Mix it up and then you do not have to worry about which is best.

Guideline #7: Eat just enough and avoid overeating.

"My doctor told me I had to stop throwing intimate dinners for four unless there are three other people." —Orson Welles

Make sure you are eating regularly to keep your blood sugar balanced.

And make sure you are not overeating. *Oh boy,* you are probably thinking, *this is getting complicated.* Not really. It is pretty simple—if you are eating per the guidelines above, and you are gaining weight, then you are eating more than your body needs.

It is impossible for me to say exactly how much you need because there are so many factors that play into it; how much activity you do in a day, what type of exercise you do, what food choices you are making, etc.

A general rule is to eat small meals regularly. I find that as we age, we actually need smaller portion sizes than when we are young and growing.

Need some tips for succeeding at eating smaller portion sizes?

- Use smaller bowls and plates. The size of the dish can make all the difference in the world.
- Before you take seconds, wait at least 10 minutes, so the food you have eaten has time to reach your belly and your brain has time to register that it is in there.
- When eating out at a restaurant that serves large portions, split meals or ask for a to-go box upfront and put half the food away right off, so you will not be tempted to eat it all. There is nothing loving about overstuffing your body. It creates all kinds of problems for your system.

Take these steps to not overeat and you will be doing a lot to support your health.

Guideline #8: Change where you shop.

Although my general recommendations for shopping are to do the bulk of it at farmers markets, supermarkets do play an important role in our food. When you make a change from one kind of store to another, you may find the transition easier if you do it gradually.

If you currently shop at large supermarket chains and warehouse stores, try changing to major health food chains.

If you currently shop at major health food chains, try switching to smaller co-op style health food stores.

If you currently shop at smaller co-op health food style stores, add in the farmers markets and consumer supported agriculture clubs or CSAs.

Guideline #9: Change where and how often you eat out.

In Los Angeles, we are very lucky. Finding restaurants that sell food that is direct from farm to table is pretty easy. Likewise, you can find restaurants all over this city that sell grass-fed meats and organic produce. I realize that that is not the case all over this country. However, if you look up on the Internet for restaurants that sell grass-fed meats and organic vegetables, or farm-to-table restaurants, the chances are you may find some. If organic is not available, then choose a restaurant where they make everything in-house—you won't believe what is in commercial salad dressings.

Regardless, if you are in a big city with lots of food options or not, let's face it, when you eat out, you are never really going to know exactly what you are eating. That is why I suggest that you prepare more food for yourself. When you cook at home, you know exactly what you are getting. You are also making sure the food is fresh and handled in clean ways. Not to mention the money you will be saving.

Guideline #10: Travel wisely; travel prepared…Secrets to traveling and eating healthy.

When you travel, there is one secret to doing it in a way that is healthy: Prepare ahead! Because I was unable to rely on finding food when I traveled, I have become somewhat of an expert on how to do it without eating a single thing that is not good for me. On airplanes, I always bring all my food and have for a long time. Some years ago, before I knew about chemicals and food, I was on a flight from New York to Los Angeles. I had ordered the beef plate. When it arrived, the beef was literally fluorescent orange and green. It was the craziest thing. I had no idea what they had done to it to make it that color, but even at 18, I knew it wasn't natural and didn't eat it. That was the last time I ordered meat on a plane.

When I was flying internationally during my vegetarian days, I ordered the vegan special meal. When it arrived at my seat, I could not even tell what food group it came from let alone what it was. I asked my neighbors if they had any idea and neither one could tell either. That was it for me. I just stopped eating airplane food from that day on and have carried my own food when I fly.

Post 9/11, a few things have changed. You cannot bring creamy foods such as hummus or salad dressing, unless it is under 3.4 ounces, through security. So, I make chunky avocado bruschetta instead of guacamole, for example. I take the small packets of organic nut butter you can buy at most health food stores instead of larger ones. I bring whole or cut up vegetables. Sliced organic lunch meats keep nicely as well. You cannot carry ice or ice packs through security, so I bring a baggie and get ice on the other side of security. Most of the fast food chains have ice machines with their soda dispensers, or I just ask for a couple of extra large cups of ice. I also make sure I have enough food for delayed flights and I even carry something for my first meal when I arrive at my destination. That gives me plenty of time to find a health food store or appropriate restaurant in the area.

Also, when traveling, I always look up my available food options before I go. Before I arrive at a place, I already know what is available, and already have my plans for how I will get there. I know, for many of you, this may sound extreme, but when you remember the number of chemicals in a single Burger King Milk Shake, it may help motivate you. Imagine the amount of chemicals you would be eating if you ate three meals in a day at convenience restaurants.

If you have food sensitivities, such as gluten intolerance, and will be traveling to a foreign speaking country, I recommend you print out something that says, "I have a _____ Allergy" before you go (In this case, I call it an allergy. It is a much more universally understood idea). Doing this small thing takes a whole lot of stress off traveling abroad.

I recently took a trip to Europe and visited three different countries. I had my printouts for each country. Even though I almost never needed them, it was a great peace of mind to know I had them if I did.

Guideline #11: Everything in moderation is okay.

If you do not have an allergy or an intolerance to a substance, then anything in moderation is okay as long as it is a food.

This also covers alcohol and coffee.

The tricky part with substances that are addictive like alcohol and coffee is to keep your relationship a healthy one.

Oh, the love affair we have with coffee. For many, there is nothing like that hot morning pick-me-up. And yet, drinking coffee or caffeine every day can have its detriments.

The problem with coffee and any other caffeine source used every day is this: when you drink a stimulant every morning or, worse, several times a day, you are giving up something that is very important. You are giving up your ability to know how you actually feel. Even if you drink coffee because you "just love the flavor," you are unfortunately falling victim to its drug-like effect on the body.

Coffee and/or caffeine have many effects on your body. It affects your heart, your brain, your digestion. It is a diuretic, causing you to lose fluids. Coffee can raise blood pressure, and it causes adrenal or stress hormones to be released into your system.

When you drink something that has a drug-like effect on the body, you lose your ability to know how you actually feel. If you are tired, then it is a really good idea to know that you are tired. Without that information, it is impossible to know that your body is having a problem and needs some attention.

If you were riding a tired horse, would you keep kicking it to get it to go faster? You wouldn't if you valued having a horse to ride. Everyone knows that if you overwork a tired horse, it will eventually go lame, or worse, collapse. Why then is it okay to kick your body into action every day if not several times a day by drinking a stimulant?

I understand that getting up and going in the morning may feel more important than the long-term effects of having a balanced relationship with caffeine, but needing caffeine every day is no different than any other quick fix. It isn't a lasting solution to the fatigue you are feeling, and, in the long term, it will not support you in your goal of vital health.

If you get a headache when you do not have your morning cup of Joe, then I can guarantee you are having an unhealthy relationship to caffeine.

By developing a balanced relationship to caffeine, having it as a treat no more than 3-4 days a week, you are going a long way to making sure your body stays balanced and healthy.

Try adding variety to your morning ritual. If you are a daily caffeine drinker, then start decreasing the amount you have slowly. When your body is ready, try adding other things to your morning routine. Try drinking green or other organic herbal tea in the mornings. Have some hot water with lemon. This not only gets the circulation going, it also helps the liver detoxify. Or here's an idea: make yourself a raw cacao hot chocolate for a yummy morning wake-up drink.

I am not saying never have coffee. However, when you wake up in the morning, rather than just grabbing the closest cup, take a minute to check in and see how you feel. Ask yourself what would be the most supportive choice you could make. I am not suggesting you give it up completely; I am just suggesting that, for your long-term health, you keep coffee as an occasional lover instead of your co-dependent friend.

Everything I just said about coffee can be applied to alcohol, although alcohol is not a stimulant, but rather a depressant. If you are drinking it every day, it is likely that you have developed a dependence on it. I know there is a big debate about whether regular alcohol consumption is good for your health. Much of the evidence supports that it may be; however, the clients I see in my clinic who drink a couple of glasses of wine a day all seem to share one thing in common, a stressed out liver. Take the alcohol away for a while and the liver improves.

So, no, I am not saying you cannot have a glass of wine, but I am suggesting that you choose to maintain a balanced relationship with alcohol. If you are drinking it every day, ask yourself why? If it helps you relax, then add some other things into your nightly routine that will actually decrease the stress on your system such as taking a walk after work or a hot bath before bed. Instead of relying on a substance every day that ultimately will increase the stress on your body by giving your liver more work to do, incorporate new habits that will actually decrease your stress level.

END NOTES

1. "How to Combine Food to Make Complete Protein," accessed August 29, 2015, http://www.wikihow.com/Combine-Food-to-Make-Complete-Protein

CHAPTER 8

Making the Transition

Nobody can go back and start a new beginning, but anyone can start today and make a new ending.—Maria Robinson

Change Isn't Always Easy but You Are Really Worth It.

For some people, learning something new comes very easily. However, for most of us, learning something new can feel stressful, especially when it affects the routines of our daily lives. Nothing affects our daily routine more than making dietary changes. I remember when I was a vegetarian, and several health practitioners said I had to eat meat; I was at a complete loss for how to do that. After all, I had been abstaining from meat for 15 years. When, at one point in my healing it was suggested I stop eating meat, I went into a panic, "What am I going to eat?" I exclaimed.

After I calmed down, I laughed at myself remembering that for 15 years, I managed not to eat meat and I was sure I could do it again. The same thing happened when, after 10 years of avoiding dairy, I added it back into my diet for just a few months. When another healthcare practitioner suggested I stop, I felt like crying. I couldn't fathom what I was going to eat without my raw cheese. Then again, I had to remind myself that I had chosen not to eat dairy for 10 years in the past; I could do it again.

If you feel overwhelmed as if you just cannot succeed at making dietary changes, the first thing to do is stop and take a deep breath. You are not alone. Most people feel this way when faced with a big change. Change takes time and commitment; however, in this case, the rewards you will receive from that time and commitment will pay you back in more ways than you can imagine right now.

As one of my mentors says, "People will never know what we have done for them; they will never know the diseases they do not get." Likewise, by making these dietary changes, you will never know what health challenges you have avoided. But isn't avoiding a health crisis worth the risk of being uncomfortable in the short run?

The reason I suggest you start with the The 21-Day Diet Detox is that, although the change gradient is steep at first, in the end, it makes the transition much easier. While making this transition, it will be helpful if you remember a few important truths.

Truth #1: Feeding yourself well is ultimately an act of self-love.

Growing up, I was often plagued with an overall feeling of discontent and, at times, downright sadness. When I would share my feelings with people, they would look at me with care and say, "You just need to love yourself."

Nothing got my ire up faster than being told, "You just need to love yourself." Someone who is in the middle of a chaotic life born out of a lack of self-love does not have the tools to love herself! Telling someone to do so is as realistic as telling someone who has never played the piano to play a Mozart concerto.

In my personal experience, backed up by watching the majority of people with whom I've worked, when you are not able to feel love for yourself, you can't just turn it on because someone says it is a good idea.

Of course, it's a good idea! The how of it is another story.

Learning to love oneself is a journey that requires dedication, focus, and introspection. However, I have a secret to share, a secret that took me years to realize.

When you care for something or someone, truly care, you will eventually fall in love.

If you find a mangy sick stray puppy with sores all over its body from fleas and mites and you make the decision to bring it home, you may not be feeling all that loving at first. It may even feel like a major pain in your neck, especially when it poops all over, keeps you up at night, and generally disrupts your schedule.

But over time, as you continue to care for it, something starts to happen. It begins to behave a little better, it becomes a little more self-reliant, and, one day, you wake up and find you actually love the little bugger. Furthermore, you can't even imagine how you ever didn't. It is inevitable. Over time, as you care for something or someone, love is what happens.

Right now, you may not be feeling so loving towards your body. It may be causing you pain. You may feel sick or have some disease you are living with. You may feel fat or unattractive. You may feel cranky, angry, or depressed.

Loving your body, let alone yourself may feel like an insurmountable challenge. When you don't love yourself, then taking care of yourself, making yourself a priority can feel impossible. In the beginning, it may take some conscious effort and maybe a little willpower, but don't give up!

Do it long enough, and I promise you will start to feel better. As your moods improve, liking yourself becomes easier. You may start to act nicer, your anger may decrease. After a while, you'll find the love seeping through. It's inevitable. And once the love is there, making choices that are not in support of your well-being become difficult, if not impossible.

Eating well, taking the time to buy and prepare food that is nourishing, and choosing restaurants that serve food that is chemically clean and rich in nutrition are all acts of care. Making sure when you go to a party or are traveling that you have a plan in place to assure you do not have to feel deprived or eat things that are harmful to you are all acts of self-care.

If you need to, *fake it* in the beginning! Fake that you like yourself. Go through the motions of taking care of yourself. As you make yourself and your health a priority, a little bit of self-love will start to shine through. What felt like an effort when you began will become second nature.

Truth #2 Changing habits may not always be easy; it is, however, always attainable.

"You haven;t failed until you quit trying." Gordon B. Hinckley

What and when you eat is just a habit, like many other habits. It was learned, usually over a lifetime. Many of the habits we have are what I call nonnegotiable habits. Nonnegotiable habits are those habits you would never think of going without. Smoking cigarettes for many is a nonnegotiable habit, but even if you do not smoke cigarettes, I guarantee you have some nonnegotiable habits. And all habits, even nonnegotiable ones, can be changed. The question is do we want to enough?

Everyone has "must do, nonnegotiable" habits. For some, skipping that morning coffee is not an option. For others, making sure they brush their teeth, shower, and put on make-up before exiting the house is a nonnegotiable. For others, going a day or two without exercise is unthinkable.

What are yours? What are the things you just "would **not**" go without doing in a day?

Feeding yourself well can also become a nonnegotiable for you. Eating nutritious chemical-free food can be a daily habit in your life. So much so, that you wouldn't even think of doing anything else.

Right! You might be saying, "That is just not going to happen." Well, if you think about it, what is the consequence of skipping your other nonnegotiable habits. If you left your makeup off for a day, what is going to happen? You might be seen by someone in your natural state. Although that may feel life threatening to some, certainly, no one has ever died from a lack of makeup.

If you skipped taking a shower for a day, you may make a few people uncomfortable with your smell, and, if it went on long enough, maybe you would jeopardize your job. But the last time I checked, not showering is not a cause of death either. If you went without brushing your teeth, you run the risk of having bad breath and maybe a few cavities or, at the worst, losing your teeth. If you skip having coffee or cigarettes, you may upset a few people with your crankiness, and may suffer headaches for a few days, but actually, you'd probably really just be doing your body some good.

However, if you keep eating chemical-laden food products, skipping meals, and/or overeating, you are heading toward health problems. Based on statistics, many of you are heading towards serious health problems and even an increased chance of early death.

Is it really an option to not make these changes?

Changing habits is not easy, but it is doable. To do so, we must apply conscious, consistent daily practice. To take you from where you are to a place where feeding yourself well is a nonnegotiable will require conscious, consistent daily practice, until you have formed new habits that do not require thinking.

When we change something we do, we are embarking on a journey of making new habits. Starting with where you are and making changes gradually goes a long way to assuring that you will sustain the changes you have made. It is often said that, for the average person, that takes about three months. From my experience, everyone is different and it is more successful to take as long as you need than to set a goal with a time frame that feels unrealistic for you. It is better to succeed slowly than to fail quickly. So, do not give up. You can do it! I know you can because I know you are worth every amount of effort it will take to succeed!

The 21-Day Diet Detox

The purpose of the 21-Day-Diet Detox is simple. By doing The 21-Day Diet Detox, you will be giving your body a vacation. Eating in a way that creates very little to no stress on the system allows your body to rest. By decreasing the internal stress your body is under, you create the environment for healing to occur.

Doing The 21-Day Diet Detox has the potential to assist you in many ways.

1. It can help you identify if the food you are eating is affecting how you feel.
2. It will help you figure out if you are gaining or carrying extra weight due to the food choices you are making.

3. It will help you identify if you have any food intolerances.
4. It will help you make the transition from a diet filled with C.R.A.P. to one filled with food.

In 21 days, you are unlikely to experience complete healing, as healing occurs over time. However, by changing what you eat, you will be creating the foundation for healing to occur.

To experience the benefits of The 21-Day Diet Detox, you will be eating food that supports your body in healing by providing a variety of nutrient-rich clean food, and eating in a way that balances your blood sugar. Simultaneously, you will be avoiding foods that are likely to cause inflammation, foods that have a high chance of being an intolerance, and as many chemicals as possible. Do this and you will have less stress on your body.

What you will eat to achieve this depends on how you are currently eating. Since changing the way you eat will cause a natural detoxification or systemic cleansing to occur, you want to make changes on a gradient that will be both sustainable for you and gentle enough from how you currently eat for you to be successful. In other words, you want to improve on how you eat now, without being too drastic.

Remember the goal is to decrease stress on your body—a drastic change will increase stress.

Choose the level that is right for you.

There are three levels. Make sure to choose the level that will be different than your daily routine and yet manageable for you to maintain for the full 21 days.

Level 3 Diet Detox

Do you
- ✓ Eat out often
- ✓ Eat fast food weekly
- ✓ Drink coffee daily
- ✓ Alcohol regularly
- ✓ Take any medications or hormones

✓ Drink sodas
✓ Use artificial sweeteners
✓ Eat foods and use products with chemicals in them without concern

If so, then the kindest thing you can do for your body is the Level 3 Diet Detox.

This level will allow your body to make big strides towards healing while transitioning at an appropriate pace. This should help you to avoid experiencing uncomfortable symptoms.

Remember stress hinders healing. It is less stressful, and more sustainable for your body to make changes gradually over time than to do them drastically all at once. Likewise, if you are thin and do not want to lose weight, or have a more serious health challenge, then the Level 3 is the best choice for you.

Level 2 Diet Detox

If you usually do the following, you will have the best results from the Level 2 Diet Detox :

✓ Prepare a good portion of your food at home
✓ Eat vegetables regularly
✓ Also eat pasta, bread and other processed food regularly
✓ Drink alcohol several days a week
✓ Drink coffee more often than not

Level 1 Diet Detox

If you tend to do the following, then Level 1 Diet Detox is your best choice:

✓ Eat organic food sometimes
✓ Shop at healthier large chain stores
✓ Use coffee and alcohol sparingly
✓ Desire to lose weight

The difference between the three levels is mainly how many solid meals versus liquid meals you eat in a day.

Which level is best for you? Check the boxes that apply to you.

Level 1	Level 2	Level 3
Eat mostly at home	Prepare a good portion of your food at home, eat out a few days a week	Eat out often Eat fast food weekly
Organic vegetables are your friend	Eat vegetables regularly, organic sometimes	Vegetables?
Processed food is a treat rather than the norm	Also eat pasta, bread and other processed food regularly	Most of your food comes from a box or is pre-made
Use coffee and alcohol sparingly	Drink coffee more often than not. Drink alcohol several days a week	Drink coffee daily & alcohol regularly
Consider yourself generally healthy	Have a few health concerns	Have a health challenge or take medications or hormones daily
Drink primarily water	Drink a variety of drinks	Drink sodas regularly
Never use artificial sweeteners	Occasional artificial sweetener use	Use artificial sweeteners regularly
Diligent about chemical exposure as much as possible	Try to avoid chemicals most of the time	Do not really think about chemicals

Count the checks in each level. The level that is right for you is the level you checked the most boxes in. If there is an even number of checks, go with the level you feel you are most likely to succeed at.

What You Will Be Avoiding and Why

Regardless of which level you choose, you will be avoiding all of the food and foodstuff listed below, with the exceptions noted for Level 3.

1. **Avoid foods that are common food intolerances.**

Avoiding potential food intolerances decreases stress on your system and will help you identify what, if any, foods are problematic for your body when you transition off the Challenge.

Food intolerances can be a major source of stress on the body. The foods listed below are the most common food intolerances. When consumed daily, food intolerances are often difficult to identify. By avoiding these foods 100 percent for 3 weeks and introducing them one at a time while monitoring weight and symptoms, you will be able to determine which, if any, foods are causing stress to your system. If you do the Diet Detox and do not remove all food intolerances, you are likely to **not** experience the full benefits.

Dairy (all milk, cheese, butter, yogurt and other milk by products)	Grains (except on level 3)
Eggs	All Soy products
Nuts and Seeds (except hemp and flax, and pumpkin seeds)	Protein powders
Gluten	Corn products

2. **Avoid foods that create extra work for the liver and your adrenals.** Doing this decreases the workload on the organs that play a crucial role in the detoxification process.

Caffeine	All chemical additives
Alcohol	Heated oils
Artificial sugar	Most oils except those listed below

3. **Avoid all foods that can promote inflammation in the body.**
Inflammation is a major cause of almost all disease processes.

The following foods can increase inflammation in the body. One of the purposes of the Diet Detox is to decrease inflammation in your system.

Potato	Pork
Eggplant & other nightshades	Hot spices (e.g., chilies & hot sauce)
All added sugar	Citrus fruit (except lemons & lime)
Red meat (except where indicated)	

Avoid taking a lot of supplements and vitamins unless they are prescribed by a licensed healthcare provider.

In many cases, clients come in and are taking so many supplements that their liver and kidneys are overworking. The nature of cleansing, even natural cleansing, increases the work for the liver and kidneys. It is best to avoid all self-prescribed supplements while doing the The 21-Day Diet Detox, as it will naturally support your body to cleanse.

Especially avoid supplements and green powders containing chlorella and spirulina. Chlorella and spirulina are great detoxifiers. However, even when taken in small amounts, they can increase the level of detoxification so much that it overloads the system. They are strong medicine, and, in my opinion, they should **only be consumed** when under the supervision of a health care practitioner.

What You Will Be Eating

Regardless of the Diet Detox you choose, you will:

1. Eat as many vegetables from the "unlimited vegetables list" as you like.

2. Eat no less than four 1-cup servings from the unlimited vegetables list per day. More is preferred (raw, juiced, water sautéed, steamed, or as soups). Vegetable consumption must include two boiled vegetables daily.

3. Eat no more than 3-4 servings of fruit a day from the list provided. Less is okay.

4. Eat 3-4 oz. servings of animal protein or a 6 oz. serving of fish protein 1 to 3 times a day, cooked without oil (frequency depends on the level you choose).

5. Consume no less or more than 3-4 tablespoons of added organic cold-pressed unheated oils per day from list provided only (added to shakes, poured over food, or added in soups after they have been cooked only).

6. Celtic and or Himalayan Sea Salt daily, as much as you crave.

7. Add herbs and non-hot spices such as dill, basil, thyme, oregano, parsley, cilantro, as desired.

8. Hemp and flax, and pumpkin seeds in shakes

Approved Foods for all 3 levels of the Diet Detox

1. **Unlimited Organic Vegetables List** (no less than four 1-cup servings a day)

Artichoke	Celery	Leafy Greens
Asparagus	Chard	Lettuce
Beets	Cilantro	Leeks
Bell Peppers (avoid w/ pain)	Collards	Mustard Greens
Bok Choy	Cucumber	Onions
Broccolli, broccolini & Broccoflower	Dandelion greens	Parsley
	Green peas	Pumpkin
Brussels Sprouts	Green beans	Radishes
Cabbage	Kale	Seaweed; Nori, Hijiki, Wakame from low radiation area
Carrots	Kabocha squash	
Cauliflower	Tomatoes (avoid w/pain)	
Spaghetti squash	Yellow squash	Zucchini
Spinach		
Sprouts, Green		

Approved Organic Fruit (in quantities listed)
No more than 3-4 servings a day

½ Avocado	Red Grapes 1 cup	Plums- 2 pitted
½ Bananas green-tipped	Kiwi 1	Pomegranate 1/2 cup
Blackberries (1 cup)	Lemons	Raspberries 1 cup
Blueberries (1 cup)	Limes	Rhubarb 2 cups
Cherries (I cup)	Papaya 1 cup cubed	Strawberries ½ cup
Cranberries 1 cup (unsweetened)	Peaches 1 medium	
	½ Pear	
Fuji or green apples ½ Medium		

Organic Free-Range Animal Protein
3-ounce servings per non-liquid meal

Chicken	Turkey	Duck

Or Wild-caught low-mercury and low-radiation fish
6-ounce servings per non-liquid meal*

Salmon	Sardines packed in olive oil

*Check the Internet to see which fish are available in your area that are wild caught, and low in mercury and radiation. Or you can order from a supplier, at the writing of this book my favorite is vitalchoice.com, which tests for both mercury and radiation levels in the fish they sell.

4. No less or more than 3-4 tablespoons of a variety of organic, cold-pressed unheated oils per day.

Olive oil	Sesame oil
Coconut oil	Walnut oil

Beverages

Purified Water, 6 to 10 eight-oz glasses a day	Water w/ Organic Frozen Berries
Green Tea steeped 1 minute or less	Pellegrino - limited amounts
Herbal Tea	

Level 1: The 21-Day Diet Detox Guidelines

This is the most cleansing of the three Diet Detoxes. With the increased nutrition you will be eating, and the lightened load on the liver and digestive tract, the body will be able to naturally clean house at a deeper level. On this version of the Diet Detox, you are likely to lose the most amount of weight and eliminate the most stored toxins.

In this variation, you will be eating one solid meal, and two liquid meals a day.

I recommend you make a shake for one meal, and have one of the soup variations for the second meal. One meal a day, you will be eating 3 ounces of animal protein or 6 ounces of fish and vegetables from the list provided.

A sample of what this may look like:

1. Breakfast   Shake
2. Lunch   Protein and a salad
3. Dinner   Hot soup with avocado chunks and/or hemp seeds sprinkled on top and a little oil drizzled on top.

Note: Avocado should never be heated, as it's far too high in unsaturated fats.

Level 2: The 21-Day Diet Detox Guidelines

Eat only from the original foods lists provided
Eat two meals a day that consist of vegetables and 3 ounces of animal protein or 6 ounces of fish.

Replace your third meal with either a soup or a shake (see recipes ideas provided). Many people choose to have a shake for breakfast and eat their meals at lunch and dinner.

Level 3: The 21-Day Diet Detox Guidelines

This is the gentlest gradient of the three detox plans. However, it will still do the job. If you eat a lot of processed food in your everyday life, then you will likely lose weight on this Diet detox if that is desired. Another reason to choose this level of diet detox is if you do not desire to lose weight. If weight loss is not desired ,then adding in the beans and rice will help you maintain your weight.

On Level 3, you can add to the above food lists the following grass-fed, range-free meats to your diet 3 times a week or less.

Lamb	Venison
Bison	2 Eggs (Eggs are a very high allergen so if possible it is recommended that you leave them out)

Limited Starchy Vegetables to ½ cup total per day at most

Sweet Potato	Japanese purple sweet potato
Yams	

At most a handful of Raw Unsalted Nuts, soaked is best, but not mandatory, per day.

Raw almonds	Sunflower seeds	Pumpkin seeds

Brown Rice, Quinoa, and/or Lentils

½ cup brown rice or ¼ quinoa (that has been soaked prior to cooking) with ½ cup lentils per meal to replace the animal protein

Coffee

If you drink several cups of coffee a day, and feel that going without would be too challenging, continue to have 1 cup of organic coffee maximum per day. If you normally only drink 1 cup a day, then I recommend you either have no more than ½ cup or leave it out altogether. Coffee can add stress to your body. If your body is stressed then it will not detoxify well, and you may hinder the benefits of the Challenge.

On this level of the Diet Detox, each day you will be:

1. Making food choices from the original food lists provided plus the added foods listed above.
2. Eating three meals a day consisting of unlimited vegetables from the vegetables list, or a starchy vegetable in the amounts provided and 3 ounces of meat protein, or 6 ounces of fish protein.
3. Eating at least two snacks a day between meals consisting of vegetables from the unlimited vegetables list and/or a small handful of raw nuts from the list provided. (see soup recipes for snack ideas)

Important notes regardless of the Diet Detox you choose

You must avoid feeling hungry except right before mealtime. These are not deprivation diets. You should feel well fed, just with different foods than you are accustomed to eating. Make sure you always have a snack with you to avoid the stress of a blood sugar drop.

Remember, this is not a forced detoxification or extreme cleanse. It is 100 percent safe. All you are doing is adding more nutrients into your body and eliminating added chemicals and inflammatory foods. Because you are not taking herbs or other substances to force your body to detoxify, it will only do so if the environment is right.

Level 1	Level 2	Level 3
How They Are the Same		
No Alcohol	No Alcohol	No Alcohol
No Added sugar	No Added sugar	No Added sugar
No Chemical additives	No Chemical additives	No Chemical additives
No Potatoes & Eggplant	No Potatoes & Eggplant	No Potatoes & Eggplant
Snacks Required	Snacks Required	Snacks Required
3-4 Servings of fruit a day only	3-4 Servings of fruit a day only	3-4 Servings of fruit a day only
Unlimited Vegtables (from the list provided)	Unlimited Vegtables (from the list provided)	Unlimited Vegtables (from the list provided)
No Heated oils	No Heated oils	No Heated oils
No citrus except lemons and limes	No citrus except lemons and limes	No citrus except lemons and limes
*Unlimited Sea Salt	*Unlimited Sea Salt	*Unlimited Sea Salt
3-4 TBS. Unheated Oil per day	3-4 TBS. Unheated Oil per day	3-4 TBS. Unheated Oil per day

*unless advised by your doctor to limit due to high blood pressure or other health challenge.

Level 1	Level 2	Level 3
How They Differ		
Biggest Dietary Change	Moderate Change	Gentle Gradient Change
Largest weight loss potential	Weight loss probable	Weight loss may or may not occur
2 liquid meals a day	1 liquid meal a day	0-1 liquid meal per day
No Caffeine	No Caffeine	Limited Caffeine
No Red Meat or Pork	No Red Meat or Pork	Limited Red Meat, No Pork
No Eggs	No Eggs	Limited Eggs
No Legumes & Grains	No Legumes & Grains	Rice, Quinoa & Lentils only
No Starchy Vegetables	No Starchy Vegetables	Limited starchy Vegtables
Hemp, Flax, Pumpkin & Sunflower seeds only	Hemp, Flax, Pumpkin & Sunflower seeds only	Hemp, Flax, and Pumpkin seeds, plus other nuts permitted

Because the only thing you are doing is changing your food choices, there is no chance for the negative health challenges that can arise with stronger cleanses.

If you have a health concern and are under the care of a doctor, please share this page with them to seek their approval prior to commencing. The word cleanse can make some doctors nervous, so it is important that they understand what you actually would be doing.

Some people feel best doing a combination of the three levels. Week one they begin with level 3; week two, they do level 1; and then week three, they end with level 2. This eases the body into and out of the changes you have made.

Possible Symptoms

That said, as your body adjusts to the change, you may experience symptoms. Following are some of the common symptoms people experience.

In the first week of any of the three challenges, you may feel tired. If you do:

- Make sure you are not skipping meals.
- Make sure you are eating enough oils.
- Make sure you are eating snacks.
- Make sure you are moving your body daily.

The first few days, some people experience headaches; this can mean your liver is struggling to handle the natural detoxification that your body is doing. If this happens, support your liver by:

- Drinking warm water with lemon
- Exercising gently
- Tapping on your right rib cage
- Increase leafy green vegetables in your diet
- Try eating a small amount of dandelion greens (they are bitter)

If you suspect you are suffering from a caffeine withdrawal headache, drink ½ cup of black tea (no cream and sugar).

You may feel deprived, but that is because you have eliminated your comfort foods. Pay attention to what you are craving the most. It may help you understand your body better. Remember, nothing tastes as good as healthy feels.

What Your Cravings Can Mean

Sugar cravings

- Low blood sugar, not snacking enough
- Low serotonin levels —you may be using sugar to boost your moods

- Fatigue, you may be using sugar to give you a short energy lift

Salt cravings

- You may be experiencing low adrenals. Salt is the number one nutrient used by the adrenals to make adrenal hormones. Try increasing Celtic or Himalayan sea salt until cravings stop.
- You may be low in other essential minerals.

Protein cravings

- You may have low adrenals. Protein can boost adrenal hormones temporarily.

Coffee cravings

- Low adrenals
- Low blood sugar
- Physiological coffee addiction—should pass in 3 to 4 days

Alcohol cravings

- Low blood sugar
- Alcohol intolerance
- You need to exercise

At first, the food you are eating may taste bland to you. If it does, know that this will eventually pass.

These Diet Detoxes are designed to be bland. The reason for this is to give your taste buds a chance to rest and become resensitized. Due to the saturation of chemical flavors added to processed foodstuff, (yes, most of the flavor in processed food comes from added chemicals rather than the food itself), taste buds can lose their ability to taste as fully as they once did. As they resensitize, you will require less saturated flavors. The flavors in your food will begin to stand out more, making added sweet, salty, and spicy flavors less needed for food enjoyment.

CHAPTER 9

Sample Meals on the 21-Day Diet Detox

Breakfast & the Level 3 Diet Detox

For the level 3 Diet Detox, you will eat solid food for breakfast.

Breakfast is the meal most people struggle with changing. However, it may help you to know that breakfast preferences are learned. I first realized this when I was living in Japan. For breakfast, I was often served miso soup, fish, vegetables, and rice.

When I mention this to my clients, they often make faces, as the idea of eating such things for breakfast is a turn off to many. However, I eat vegetables and protein for breakfast almost every day. The idea of having sweets for breakfast such as donuts or pancakes is actually unappealing to me, and I do not eat eggs. Based on my personal experience, I know it is possible to enjoy breakfast without any of those foods, as breakfast is my favorite meal. As I said, taste preferences are a learned behavior, a learned behavior that can and will change, given time and consistent exposure to new flavors. To make this transition easier I have included some meal ideas that can be used as a breakfast substitute.

- 3 ounces of steak and Bieler's broth soup
- Chicken with raw vegetables
- Homemade chicken soup
- Rice with lentils and ½ avocado

- Shake
- Veggie scramble with eggs, no more than 3 times a week

Lunch or Dinner While on the Diet Detox

Lunch and dinner are often easier as we are accustomed to eating protein for lunch and dinner. Where people have trouble is in finding the time to prepare the food. The key to succeeding at this is to prepare in advance. Every day, I prepare my breakfast and lunch first thing in the morning and will often eat similar foods for the two meals that day. However, doing this means I make sure to vary what I am eating every day.

- 3 ounces of protein and a soup or salad
- 3 ounces of protein with cooked vegetables with oil or a dip
- 6 ounces of fish with soup and/or salad
- 3 ounces of protein with raw vegetables cut up and a dip

Some Soup and Shake Recipe Ideas

Regardless of the Diet Detox level you are undertaking, soups play a valuable part of the process. On the level 1 Diet Detox, soup will be a required part and can be great not only as one of your liquid meals, but also as a snack. On the Level 2 Diet Detox, you can choose between soup and a shake as your one liquid meal. On the level 3 Diet Detox, soup can always be a meal option.

However, regardless of the Detox level you are enjoying, soup can be very helpful as a snack. I often carry a glass jar with soup in it throughout my day, whether I am doing a Diet Detox or not. It is a great way to easily get nutrition in your body, since you can drink anywhere, even in a meeting without it being disruptive. Making sure you do not get hungry is an essential part of this process, so making sure you always have snacks available is essential to your success.

Bieler's Detox Soup

1 Carrot	1 Clove garlic (optional) while on the Challenge)	1 Wedge lemon without the peel
1 Avocado		2 Tbs. dulse or a pinch of sea salt
	¼ Cup parsley	
1 Tbs. raw sauerkraut or chickpea miso (not soy)	1 Cup sprouts	1 Tsp. olive oil added after it is blended
1/3 Onion	½ Cup another large sprouts	

Put 1 cup of water into a stockpot. Put the string beans in first and steam for about 5 minutes. Then put in celery and zucchini and steam for another 5- 7 minutes. Do not overcook. When done, put the water and vegetables into the blender. Blend until liquefied. Add a large handful of parsley. Blend until parsley is liquefied.

Other vegetables can be added as desired for variety. Try adding carrots, beets (cooked first), spinach, or other greens for variety. If the parsley is too strong, you can leave it out.

If you are on the Level 3 Diet Detox, you can try adding half a sweet potato for added richness.

Add Celtic sea salt at the end for flavor and serve with a table-spoon of oil; olive oil, coconut oil, and walnut oil are my favorites for richness.

Raw Soup Recipe

Great when doing a Diet Detox in spring and summer (can be used to replace a shake if a more savory meal is desired).

Mix in a blender:

1 Carrot	1 Clove garlic (optional) while on the Challenge)	1 Wedge lemon without the peel
1 Avocado		
1 Tbs. raw sauerkraut or chickpea miso (not soy)	¼ Cup parsley	2 Tbs. dulse or a pinch of sea salt
	1 Cup sprouts	1 Tsp. olive oil added after it is blended
1/3 Onion	½ Cup another large sprouts	

Hearty Miso Soup

(Can be used as a snack or a liquid meal.)

Directions

Chop a variety of vegetables into small pieces. Bok choy, chard, spinach, broccoli, are nice but any will work.

Grate carrots, zucchini, turnips, or even daikon radish.

Add 2 cups water to a pot. Place all vegetables in the water.

Bring to a boil and simmer covered until vegetables are soft.

Turn heat off. Spoon 1 scoop of water into a cup and add 1-2 tbs. of soy-free miso; stir until miso is mixed with water.

Serve vegetables and water into a large cup or bowl. Stir in miso mixture.

Beef or Bison Bone Broth

(Can be used as a snack or added to any soup for extra nourishment. Great if you have been ill, feel depleted, and/or need to rebuild on a deep level.)

Bake brown organic, grass-fed bones in the oven for best flavor. (To do so, place the bones in a 350-degree oven, give or take, until brown. This is optional.)

Directions
1. Place bones in a crockpot or soup pot.
2. Add vegetable scraps as they are available.
3. Cover bones and scraps with water: Set the water level about one-inch above the bones.
4. Add two tablespoons of raw apple cider vinegar.
5. Cover the pot and set on low (crock pot) or simmer (stove top).
6. Keep the lid slightly ajar as the broth warms up to avoid boiling. (Make sure your liquid does not boil out or you will be left with burned bones.)
7. Strain the broth about 24 hours later, some people cook even longer until bones have disintegrated.
8. Add a cup of stock to make your vegetable soup heartier.
9. Add water to the bones again and make a second batch of broth. (Keep doing this until you are tired of it, or your bones have disintegrated.)

You can also have any soup that is homemade using the approved ingredients.

21-Day Diet Detox Shake Recipes

Your shakes will consist of a protein source, a serving of fruit or two, vegetables, fiber and a fat. Protein will come from hemp seeds.

Fruit comes from the list provided above. Fat comes from coconut oil, walnut oil, or sesame seed oil and avocado. Fiber comes from flax seeds.

Protein sources for each shake must equal approximately 15-20 grams. The nuts and seeds must all be raw, organic, and soaked prior to use.

- 4 tbsp hemp hearts = 20 grams protein
- ¼ cup soaked sunflower seeds* = 7 grams protein + 3 tbsp hemp seeds=20 grams
- 1/3- cup soaked Pumpkin seeds* 12 grams + 2 tbsp hemp seeds= 22 grams

*nuts and seeds to be eaten only in shakes for the level 1 and 2 Diet Detox.

If you carry the herpes virus in your system, it is best to avoid eating nuts every day. Nuts are high in arginine and can promote a herpes outbreak.

If this is the case for you, I recommend you find a source for Standard Process' Dairy-free SP Complete Powder (sold by health-care providers only), or buy a Pea only protein powder with no fla-vorings or other added ingredients. Although I do not believe that protein powders are an ideal substitute for food, in the case of the herpes virus, it is the best option.

To the soaked nuts, seeds, or protein powder you will add 1+or-tbsp. flax seeds, more if you are constipated, less if bowels are loose, ½-1 tbsp. of oil, fruit, greens and 2 or more cups of water to desired thickness.

Basic Shake Recipe

- Nuts and seeds
- 1 tbsp or more soaked flax seeds
- ½-1 tbsp oil
- greens
- fruit
- 2 cups filtered or spring water (no water from soft sided plastic water bottles) **Greens that taste good in shakes**

Celery	Parsley	Cucumber
Romaine lettuce	Spinach	Zucchini
Kale (stems removed)	Chard	Sprouts

Fruit

Choose your fruit from the list above. A serving size is indi-cated next to the fruit. Remember, you are having only 3-4 servings a day, so if you are having 2 shakes you will need to choose recipes that do not exceed your limit, or leave a fruit out on occasion.

Always drink your shake at room temperature. If the fruit is frozen and/or the vegetables are cold, warm the water before adding it to your shake.

See below for sample shake recipes, and fruit and green ideas.

Other yummy items you can try in your shake:

- 1-2 tbs. raw cacao powder a few times a week (not cocoa powder, they are very different)
- ½ tsp. alcohol free vanilla extract, or ½ vanilla bean
- A small pinch of cinnamon powder (no sugar)

How to start:

All ingredients are placed in a blender and blended until smooth. A high-powered blender like a Vitamix or Blendtec will give you the smoothest results. For lower powered blenders, you may have better results if you do not use kale and your nuts must always be soaked. Regardless of the blender type, remove the stem of kale.

Sample Shake Recipes

- ½ Banana, 1-2 tbs. flax seeds, 4 tbsp hemp seeds, 1 zucchini, ½-cup blueberries, 1- tbs. coconut oil.
- 1/4-cup soaked sunflower seeds, 1-2 tbsp flax seeds, ½ cup blueberries, 1 banana, 2 tbsp cacao powder, dash of cinnamon, 1 tbsp coconut oil
- 4 tbsp hemp seeds, 1-2 tbsp flax seeds, ½ avocado, ½- tbs. coconut oil, ½ banana (add in cacao, cinnamon, or vanilla for added flavor)

Fruit and green combinations for you to try:

Following are some fruit combinations that have been approved for taste.

If you find the flavor unpleasant, then leave out the vegetables and add them in as your taste buds adjust. Kale has a stronger flavor and can be more difficult to digest, promoting bloating. If you suffer from this symptom, use other greens and eat your kale, a highly nutritious food, cooked only.

- 1 stalk of celery, hand full of greens, 1/2 cup blueberries, 1/2 banana
- 8 romaine lettuce leaves or other greens, 1/2 banana, ½-cup grapes,
- 6 to 8 romaine lettuce leaves or other greens, 2 apricots
- 1/2 banana, 1/2 cup blueberries, plus 6 to 8 romaine lettuce leaves
- 1/2 banana, 1/2 cup fresh or frozen strawberries, 5 kale leaves or other greens
- 1 handful of strawberries, 1 handful of spinach leaves, 1 cucumber
- 2 ripe kiwis, 1/2 banana, 3 stalks celery
- 1 small bunch of chard, 1/2 peeled apples, 1/2 banana
- 1/2 pear, 2-3 kale leaves (stems removed) or other greens, mint leaves
- 1/2 pear, a handful of raspberries, 2-3 kale leaves or other greens
- 1/2 Fuji apple, handful of strawberries, 5 kale leaves or other greens
- 1 handful of strawberries, 2 handfuls of spinach leaves
- 2 ripe kiwis, 1/2 banana, 3 stalks celery
- 1 zucchini, 1/2 peeled apple, 1/2 bannana

Combine these with your protein choice, flax seeds, and an oil of your choice, for a wide variety of shake options. Remember variety is the key to meeting all of your nutritional needs.

*Note Organic Frozen Fruit is okay to use.

If you feel bloated after the shakes, or your bowel movements slow, add in a small slice of ginger to your shake, or have your shake while drinking a cup of ginger tea.

Strategies for Succeeding at The 21-Day Diet Detox During Extra Busy Work Days

- Plan in advance.
  Plan to bring your own food.
- Make a meal plan for the week ahead of time.
- If you are having two shakes a day, drink one in the morning and one at night.
- Make your lunch and snacks the night before.
- A salad and protein are good easy-to-carry lunches.
- Salads taste better when raw vegetables such as carrots, beets, zucchini, celery root, radish, and a small amount of red onion are grated.
- Place salad dressing in a small jar, or add sea salt and olive oil at home and bring sliced lemon. Cut avocado in half and place face down in salad container to keep fresh. Scoop out of shell just prior to eating.
- Bring soup with you in a jar, put some in a coffee cup, and add a small amount hot water to warm. Drink whenever you are hungry.
- Make sure your friends and colleagues know you are doing this so they can support you!
- Ask for the support you need!
- Make yourself the priority for the next three weeks!

Shopping list for the busy days

Flax crackers

- Organic sliced lunchmeats
- Cut-up carrots, celery sticks, jicama, cherry tomatoes, zucchini sticks
- Premade dips

Transitioning Off the Diet Detox

How you transition off the 21-Day Diet Detox is very important. You may be eager to go back to everyday eating. However, it is important that you follow the guidelines below as closely as you followed the guidelines during the Challenge process.

This is important for two reasons:

1. It is important that you gently increase the workload of your organs. If you fail to do this, it is possible that your system will become overburdened and your body will be forced to store toxins as fat once again.

2. You have eliminated most of the high "allergen" foods for three weeks. You now have the opportunity to learn what foods, if any, cause stress to your system. By adding in foods one by one, you will be able to observe if they adversely affect you. **If a food does affect you, you may notice symptoms such as; mood changes, instant weight gain, bloating, bowel changes, headaches, increased pain, etc.**

Directions:

- Add in each food group, one at a time.
- Choose the order you will add them in now to support your success.
- Weigh yourself the morning before you add in a food group.
- Eat that food group 1 to 2 times a day for two to three days.
- Weigh yourself every morning and note any weight change or symptoms.
- If you notice any weight gain, even 2 lbs., or any symptoms, then stop eating that food and consider it a food you should not eat.
- If you have an increase in symptoms with a food, wait until they have subsided before adding the next food.
- If you have no symptoms, then after the two to three day trial period, you can add in the next food.

Use the following chart to track what foods you are adding and any new symptoms. This will aid you in keeping the process a conscious one. It is easy to forget and add in more than one food at a time if you do not keep track in this way. Before you start to add foods back in, decide in which order you will do so, mark that order by writing a number in the box with the # sign. I recommend adding in the foods that you are missing the most first. Each day, make sure to write your weight and any symptoms you noticed.

#	Date	Food	Symptoms & Weight Change
#		Eggs	
#		Red Meat	
#		Raw Dairy	
#		Gluten/ Grain	
#		Alcohol	
#		Nuts	
#		Sweet	

After you have completed the 21-Day Diet Detox!

After you have completed The 21-Day Diet Detox, it is important that you apply the same food consciousness as you had during the Diet Detox. Now is not the time to run out and have a junk food party. It is the time to implement the changes that will guide you for the rest of your life. This is the time you will start to form new daily habits to replace the ones you broke while on the Detox. Remember this is called the Diet Detox for a reason. You have just spent 21-days detoxifying, or cleaning up your diet. If, at this point, you do not continue to apply conscious attention, then you will most likely return to your old habits, making all the effort you applied during the Diet Detox a waste.

Here is a reminder of the core principles you will be implementing as you go:

The Food Solution Guidelines Revisited
Eliminate the stress caused by what you eat

- Eliminate chemicals in what you eat (additives, colors, & GRAS additives).
- Eliminate eating things that are low in nutrition (processed foods).
- Eliminate eating things that feed immune challenges (high sugar foods, excess alcohol).
- Eliminate fried foods or highly heated oils.
- Eliminate personal food intolerances.

Increase the nutrient density of the food you eat:

- Choose organic food (higher nutrition & less chemicals).
- Choose free-range, grass-fed meats & wild caught fish only (small growers are best).
- Choose food raised/grown as close to your home as possible.
- Buy direct from the farmer when possible.
- Eat whole food (has not been ground or was ground recently).
- Use organic unrefined cold-pressed oils stored in glass.
- Eat food prepared to enhance nutrient density (soaked or fermented).

As you start to add foods back in, make a copy of the following check sheet. Use this sheet not only to assess where you are at, but also to plan where you will go next.

Start by checking off what you already do. Then choose a few habits you will change first by placing a number next to them in the order you will change them. Once you have implemented a habit, check it off and move to the next change to be made. If you stay focused on this, you will wake up one day and be eating in an entirely new way, without struggling to do so. Make sure to place the check sheet in a place where you can see it every day such as on your refrigerator or desktop.

My suggestion is that you change a couple of the things that seem simplest to you first, and then work towards the things that feel more daunting.

Making the Transition to Food

- ☐ Eat 50% raw (more in summer, less in winter).

- ☐ Eat protein daily to support healing: low-stress life, vegetarian okay; high-stress life, animal protein is better.

- ☐ Eat organic high-quality fat in small amounts daily.

- ☐ Eat plenty of fresh organic vegetables (especially leafy greens).

- ☐ Eat low-sugar fruit (eat 3/4 vegetables to 1/4 fruit daily).

- ☐ Eat grain in small quantities.

- ☐ Eat low to no flour (low nutrition, unless fermented and freshly ground).

- ☐ Eat raw organic nuts (sprouted best, especially if they are a main protein source).

- ☐ Eat no to low gluten.

- ☐ Eat low nightshades to decrease inflammation (especially if you are in pain).

- ☐ Eat raw dairy only.

- ☐ Eat no foods with added sugar (adds empty calories that become fat & feeds bugs).

- ☐ Eat as little soy as possible (small amounts of non-GMO fermented soy only).

- ☐ Eat raw desserts (in moderation).

- ☐ Drink 7-10 eight-oz. glasses of filtered water daily (avoid plastic, pH of 7.5 is best).

- ☐ Drink no to small amounts of alcohol (empty calories, stress to the liver).

- ☐ Start each day with a 16-oz. glass of room-temperature filtered water (add lemon if constipated).

- ☐ Prepare the majority of your food at home.

- ☐ Choose a variety of drinks for your morning pleasure (make coffee an occasional friend).

CHAPTER 10

Avoiding Common Pitfalls to Success

"Of course there is no formula for success except perhaps, an unconditional acceptance of life and what it brings."— Arthur Rubinstein

Once you transition from The 21-Day Diet Detox to everyday eating, there are several things to understand that will help you not only stay committed, but also avoid getting derailed. Remember, to succeed at change requires your attention and focus in the beginning. Then once you have learned the new way, it will become as effortless a part of your life as brushing your teeth is.

It is Natural to Resist Change, Just Don't Let That Stop You

Humans are, by nature, tribal. Connection is of the utmost importance to us. So, for many, changing your eating habits to ones that make you different than your tribe, i.e., family, friends, and peers can be a huge challenge.

It is literally in our genes to feel unsafe about breaking with the tribe. In primal days, breaking with the tribe meant isolation and certain death. In later years, breaking with the norm often led to persecution, being ostracized, and, in some cases, being burned or tortured to death.

Many of us have such incidences in our DNA and family lineage. I happen to know that one of my relatives was burned at the stake for participating in the founding of a new religion. That kind of thing has got to make you think twice about your choices, right?

So when we make choices that lead us to no longer be aligned with our tribe, it can feel scary and unsafe at a level beyond our conscious knowing.

The problem is that, in today's world climate, following the norm has become life threatening. It's time to take the chance; it's time to set a new example, exhibit leadership, and develop a new path. By being a trend setter rather than a trend follower, you actually not only support your own health but also set a positive example for your tribe by raising the consciousness around the survival of our planet for generations to come.

Identify What Kind of Healer You Are

"Homeostasis: The ability of the body, or a cell to seek and maintain a condition of equilibrium or stability within its internal environment when dealing with external changes."
—Biology-online.org

Homeostasis is a function of the body absolutely necessary for its survival. The body, in all its wisdom, is always prioritizing toward survival, using what is available to create the most optimal conditions.

When the body finds its natural state of homeostasis, it does what it can to maintain that state and, as a result, can be resistant to change. Changing the way you feel physically takes time as the body goes through the process of adjusting from one homeostatic state to another.

Think about the last time you started a new exercise program. You may have found it difficult at the beginning to motivate yourself to do it. But then, at some point, you realized it had become easier, almost second nature. In fact, once you had been doing it long enough, if you missed a day or two you could feel the effects of taking a break.

The influence exercise had on your body had become part of your homeostatic state. When you stopped doing it, it felt strange because your homeostatic state had started to adjust. Continue to not do it long enough and that will become the new norm, changing your homeostatic state once again.

Understand that this adjustment from one homeostatic state to another is not a universal experience. We all experience some sort of effect but will experience the change differently. In other words, we don't all heal the same way.

Straight Shot Healers

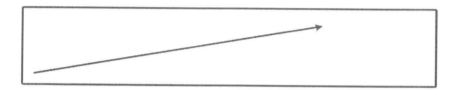

Some people are straight shot healers. Their bodies adjust to change easily, and, once pointed in the right direction, continue to feel better and better. For these people, healing is often easy and even pleasurable.

Up and Down Healers

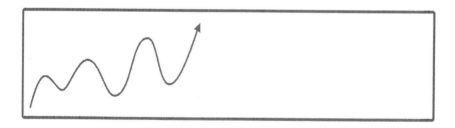

For others, the road is not so smooth. Moving from one homeostatic state to another can be fraught with a series of ups and downs, making the choice towards positive change more challenging and often requiring the support of a qualified practitioner to help them navigate the necessary changes.

I am an up and down healer. One day, I felt great and then, boom, my body would drop back into feeling bad again. For me, working with an expert practitioner was invaluable throughout my healing process.

If you are this type of healer, there are good and challenging times ahead. That is good because when you experience such extreme ups and downs, staying committed to feeling better is easier. But, at the same time, it can be challenging because it is difficult not to get discouraged during those difficult down times. However, the experience can be so extreme, giving up is not an option!

Plateau Healers

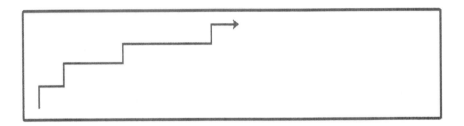

This last group often has the toughest time staying committed. The body of a plateau healer makes changes in steps and stages. When the body is taking a new step toward more optimal homeostasis you feel great, but then a frustrating plateau often follows that gain.

The times on the plateau can feel as if you are making no progress. Often an inner voice asks, "Why bother? It won't make any difference." Do not despair. If you keep your focus on improving your health, you will experience another rise.

The fact of the matter is that you are still healing; you're just not feeling or seeing the results yet. I like to think of it as the winter of your healing.

You know how in the winter, everything looks bleak, as if there isn't any life going on at all. But then, come spring, everything blossoms, bouncing back into vibrancy. Something was going on all those months; we just couldn't see it. It can be the same thing with plateau healers.

Years ago, I had an experience of this kind of healer and it left a powerful impression that has supported me and helped me support countless others on their healing journey.

At the time, recently out of acupuncture school, my co-worker was helping a family friend with her knee pain. If we learned anything in school, it was that acupuncture is great for pain.

Working on her client, my colleague was doing everything she had been taught to do for knee pain. She performed acupuncture several times a week, gave her client herbs, suggested dietary changes. Nothing was working; the knee pain was unchanged.

We sat for hours discussing her course of action, pouring over our books, looking for solutions.

Because the client was a family friend being treated for free, she kept coming, happy to support my colleague in her learning process.

After several months of this frustrating treatment, we made an unexpected discovery. The client had failed to mention when she first came in that her jaw bone was deteriorating. She was slated to have jaw surgery to replace the bone. Of course, why would she mention it? It was her knee that was bothering her, not her jaw.

During the time she was waiting for the jaw surgery, she was being treated for her knee pain. Finally, months later, when she went to her dentist for her pre-op x-rays, her jawbone had completely healed, and she no longer needed the surgery.

It turns out that in Chinese medicine, the acupuncture points and herbs used to support the knees also support the bones; they are part of the same system.

Although it seemed from a symptom point of view in terms of her knee health that nothing was happening, in actuality, her body was in a significant homeostatic change, healing on a very deep level.

Because the jaw was a greater problem for the body than the knee, the body, in all its wisdom, was healing the jaw first. Not long after she learned about her jaw being healed, her knee pain started to improve. Once the more pressing problem of the bone deterioration was solved, accompanied by her commitment to good choices, healing continued, and ultimately relieved her knee pain. That's the miraculous thing about the body—it is very wise.

If you provide your body with good things: nutrient-dense food, fresh air, clean water, easy movement, laughter, and love, it will take that good and change it's homeostatic state to a more efficient one that enhances your overall survival.

And, in its ultimate wisdom, if you feed the body food void of nutrients or underuse or overuse it, it will also take those factors and create the best possible homeostatic state, which is obviously not going to be very high on the health meter. You've heard the expression, *you get what you give?* Well, it's also true when it comes to your body's homeostasis.

And the sad part is that you may never realize you could feel any better than you do now until you are faced with a health crisis of some sort, as your body drops to a new low level of homeostasis.

When you hear about a "perfectly healthy" person who suddenly drops dead one day, you are hearing about someone who experienced the unfortunate end result of this deterioration.

Do not be lulled into a false sense of security by the fact that you are feeling "okay," even though you don't take such good care of yourself.

You may be in a low level of homeostasis. Make no mistake; if you are doing things that are <u>not</u> in support of a healthy body, they are having an effect. You may not know what that effect is until one day you wake up and find you no longer feel well, go to the doctor, and are given a diagnosis.

What Homeostatic State Are You Living In?

Are you in a low level, merely trying to survive? Or are you in an optimal level that allows you to thrive?

As I said, changing your homeostatic state can take commitment. The body's innate tendency is to return to the homeostatic state it is currently used to. Do not get discouraged. Keep making the choices that support optimal health and your body will rise to the next level. Once there, you will have a difficult time imagining how you were ever willing to settle for being anywhere else. And as one of my colleagues loves to say "you will never know the diseases you didn't get as a result."

It's Natural to Want What We Can't Have.

How many diet books are on your bookshelves right now? Have you tried all of them? Some of them? Have you tried the latest fad diet? And how many of those diets have been successful for you…long term? How many of you have gone back to your old habits regaining the weight you lost…and maybe even more, losing the vibrancy you gained when you shed the pounds, seemingly forgetting everything you learned or, worse yet, remembering it but beating yourself up for not being able to stay focused?

Any of this sound familiar? Why is this? Why is it that even if we *know* what we should do, it's so hard to do it?

It is a very human response to want what we cannot or should not have, particularly if someone else is telling us we can't have it. It is so much a part of our psyche that no matter how evolved we are, we all have, at one time or another, felt its alluring effects.

If you've ever spent time around a 2-year-old, you have seen this in action. Tell a 2-year-old to stay away from a hot stove and suddenly, no matter how many toys are around, that stove is the most interesting thing in the room.

If you've ever had a love relationship end, not by *your* choosing, that person who you maybe didn't even really like so much suddenly becomes your perfect mate. It doesn't matter if you were planning on breaking up with them, were miserable in the relationship, or just plain didn't like them. The fact that they are rejecting you suddenly makes them overwhelmingly desirable.

Let's turn our attention to our food choices with this natural response mechanism in mind. Knowing a particular food isn't "good" for you and you "shouldn't" eat it gives that food untold powers over you. Tell yourself you can't have something, and POW, your cravings intensify. And let someone else say you can't have it and Kazam! Now, you *gotta* have it!

Okay. So, you're human like the rest of us. Don't fret about it. There is another way.

Make Choices Instead of Doing "Shoulds"

Choice: Act of choosing; the voluntary act of selecting or separating from two or more things that which is preferred; the determination of the mind in preferring one thing to another; election.[1]

Should: Used to indicate obligation, duty, or correctness, typically when criticizing someone's actions: "He should have been careful."[2]

In my practice, when I intensified my focus on nutrition, I witnessed people struggling with making nutrition choices that would support health in their bodies. This struggle confused me. I assumed if they *knew* what was good for them, they would just do it. I was wrong. Knowing what they *should do* wasn't enough. As a matter of fact, knowing what they *should* do was often part of the problem.

It was perplexing to me why someone would do something they knew was harmful, particularly if they didn't feel well after doing it. Eager to understand this conundrum, I started thinking about my clients, particularly the ones who seemed to have trouble staying on track.

Sitting with a client one day, going over a long list of things she couldn't do and foods she couldn't have due to her particular food intolerances, I noticed something interesting. As we talked about how many foods were bad for her and the negative effects that would result from her eating them, I saw her shrinking away from all the restrictions in her life.

I literally saw her life force, her light, getting smaller. And I thought to myself, *this is not okay!* The whole reason for healing is so our life force can get larger, not smaller.

I began to wonder, *why is this different for me? You see, part of my health challenge involves multiple food intolerances, so the diet that is best for me leaves out many of the common foods other people enjoy. Why is making choices that avoid certain foods easy for me, and yet so difficult and painful for so many of my clients? Why don't I feel like I'm missing out, or being restricted, or punished, as they often communicate they do?*

I realized that looking at it from the perspective of restrictions, "You can't have this!" "You shouldn't do that!" I would feel pretty bad about it too. Why didn't I? Why was it that living without all those "things" didn't feel restrictive to me? And why did it feel restrictive to so many others?

During the height of my illness, I spent many years not feeling well. My energy was low. I was in constant pain and my body was under continuous stress. The choices I made every day were imperative to my well-being.

If I chose to eat one particular food that didn't agree with my body, I would literally end up in bed the next day, barely able to function. Making choices that were good for me became easy because the consequences of not doing so were so negative.

Once I experienced what was bad for my body and had to deal with those consequences, I readily stopped doing it. It was really easy.

My reasons for making the choices I made were very clear to me. I knew I wanted to wake up and feel as good as I possibly could. I knew if I didn't heal my body, I could be in serious trouble in the future.

I was choosing to feel good instead of eating that piece of bread or drinking that glass of wine. Not that those things are intrinsically bad; they just were not good for my body.

My priority was to feel good. My health was far more important to me than feeling like I was a part of the group by following their food and drink choices. As a matter of fact, saying no to alcohol allowed me to be more a part of the group because it supported me in being well enough to be out of bed and out with friends.

It suddenly hit me. I did not feel restricted because I was making a choice. I was choosing to refrain from alcohol, not because I shouldn't drink it, but because it supported my vision of a healthier me.

We are always making choices in life. Whether we enjoy the end result of that choice or not, we are still doing it because we are choosing to.

Even the person who goes to a job every day that she doesn't like does so because she is choosing to have a roof over her head and her job affords her that result. So even if she is going to a job she doesn't care for, it beats the alternative of becoming homeless and living in the street. She is making a choice.

Most of us are very clear that living in the street is not an option, so we do what we *must* to keep a roof over our heads. Even though we may not enjoy the process, we still do it by choice.

Imagine if you went in every day and felt grateful for the job you have because it is keeping a roof over your head. How would that change your experience?

When it comes to your health, choosing to place extra time and attention on the food you eat is a choice that has great reward. Getting to a new level of vitality will take time. But during that time, remembering why you are making the choices you make will make staying with it a lot easier.

Here are some simple steps to help you become more conscious of making choices that result in a positive experience. Keep this list close to help you remember that you always have a choice!

- Define your vision. Be clear about why you are doing what you are doing.
- Educate yourself about what will support you in obtaining that vision.
- Identify and evaluate your current choices and see how they do or do not support your vision.
- Put those choices into action on a daily basis and stick with them long enough to see results.
- Change your language to support the actions you are taking. For example, *I choose to go to work.* Not, *I have to go to work.* Or, *I choose to eat an apple because it supports me in feeling good.* Instead of, *I shouldn't eat that piece of cake because it will make me fat.*
- Celebrate your successes, large and small by acknowledging yourself with positive uplifting rewards.

Be Clear About Your Goal

It is impossible to be an active part of creating your dream future unless you know what that dream is.

For some people, the dream is to live to 100 and to have climbed Mt. Everest for their 80th birthday celebration. For others, it may be living in peace with sound body and mind and passing in their sleep at 89.

I hear you asking, "Why do I even need to be thinking about this?" Here's the thing: health isn't something that happens by accident. Yes, good genes can help, but, in today's world, good genes can be completely overridden by our lifestyle choices.

Making a Plan for Your Health is the Greatest Gift You Can Give Yourself and Your Family

Without your health, everything is more difficult if not downright impossible. Ask anyone who has dealt with illness. It can rob you of almost everything.

Many of us plan diligently for our financial future, but rarely have a concrete, outlined vision for the health of our physical body or what we need to do to achieve that. You can have all the money in the world, but without your health, it will do you no good. If you are diagnosed with Alzheimer's, your money may help pay for your care, but it isn't going to stop your brain from deterioration.

Life holds many unforeseen experiences. You may save and plan for your financial security, and something can come along that derails all your plans. By the same token, you may also plan your health future, and something unexpected can come along even though you "did everything right."

However, I guarantee that if you have been planning for a solid financial future, educating yourself, applying focused attention for your financial well-being, you are going to have a much better chance of recovering if the worst were to happen.

The same is true when it comes to your health. If you wait until you are sick, to learn how to be well, you are already at a deficit. And, as one who has been down that road, staying healthy is a whole lot easier and less expensive than trying to get well once you are sick.

So, the first step to better health is to create a vision of a healthy robust you, now and in the future. When we create a health vision, we can develop a health plan and make sure our vision and choices are in alignment with that plan. If you don't have a health vision, you will never know if your choices are in alignment with that vision.

I recommend that people write out a health plan for five years down the road, end of life, and somewhere in the middle. Really explore the terrain. Look deep inside and see the dream for your health future.

This will help you develop a plan of action based in reality.

If you desire to climb a big mountain in celebration of your 80th birthday, your preparations and choices will be vastly different than if your goal is to be an active grandparent enjoying the bridge club.

One dream is not better than another, just different. And they need to be treated as such so, one day, near the end of your life, you will be able to reflect and say, "That was a life well lived!"

Focus on What You Want Rather than What You Don't Want

My crazy friend Jack said to me one day, "I'm going to increase my experience of joy!"

"Good for you!" I said, thinking, *Yeah, right! Good luck with that!*

I love Jack dearly, but, by his own admission, he is a little crazy. And I was quite certain you couldn't increase your joy because you say you are going to.

Well, color me wrong! Over the next six months, I watched him do exactly that. I witnessed him get happier and happier and happier as he focused on everything that brought him joy. It was a powerful reminder of one of the laws of the universe; we get what we expect to get.

You can walk into a room and see 20 things you like about it and 20 things you don't like. But here's the secret: the things you focus on will determine your experience.

You can focus on the things you like, the things you find beautiful, things that make you feel good, or you can focus on the things that bother you, which will take you right to your "not happy" place. The choice is yours. And it **is** a choice.

In fact, in every moment, we are faced with choices, and the ones we make will determine our experience. We can see everything as being in our favor, or we can perceive everything as not in our favor. In other words, we either see the glass half full or half empty.

By focusing on the fullness present in the glass and how you might fill it further, you have a much greater chance of ending up with a full glass. If you focus instead on the emptiness of the glass and all the ways the glass is getting emptier, you will end up with an empty glass.

Your Choice Today Will Affect Your Experience Now and in the Future

And here's some good news. Your brain is equipped to support you in making this easier. It literally develops a stronger affinity toward those things we do a lot. In other words, whatever you put into practice, you will see the effects of that practice. The more we do or think something, the easier that thing becomes to do, or think about.

We train our brains to support us in focusing on that which we focus on. If we focus on things that give us pleasure, we are strengthening the brain's ability to focus on and experience pleasure. The opposite is also true. Focus on negativity and you will experience less than desirable results.

You can literally support your brain to develop neural pathways that form the habit of focusing on something you want. But here's the thing: the brain functions like a muscle. And, like any muscle, in order for it to work optimally, you have to train it.

Here's where the manifestation of your choice comes in to play. If you build the muscle of your brain that focuses on what's wrong or on the things you don't want, you will manifest the things you don't want. But if you train your brain to see what's good and what you do want, making choices that support that positive attitude, then that is what you will get.

With this in mind, I'd say it's time to get to the positive focus gym!

Change Your Language, Change Your Life

Every day we make choices. Whether those choices have positive or negative consequences, they are still choices. As mentioned earlier, you may go to a job you're not crazy about but you are choosing to go there. You also have the choice of what attitude you take when you go there. The language you use in your head and out loud helps to determine your experience.

When we shift our perspective to include this reality, we will discover the immense power of language.

By owning the choices you make and the reasons that motivate them, you will begin to realize you are not a victim to your circumstances. No matter what, you always have choice in life.

When you adopt this attitude, life opens up. If I realize I am choosing to go to my job to put a roof over my head, that might lead me to the realization that there is another job I might enjoy more that will do the same thing.

This is where the language you use becomes really important.

Even your self-talk is a huge factor in your experience. Thinking to yourself, *I have to go to work today,* can make you feel like a victim. Try it. Can't you just feel the heaviness and dread? Now think to yourself, *I choose to go to work today.* Don't you feel a bigger sense of your own powerful force?

The language around food choices you make is equally as powerful. "I choose to eat _____ instead of that sugary dessert," is a much more empowered statement than, "I'm not supposed to have that; I'm on a diet." Likewise, "Yes, I'd love some dessert," rather than "I shouldn't but I will anyway," is also a more positive statement. Guilt has a much worse effect on the body than a piece of cake ever will.

I really encourage you to watch the language you use. Every time you choose language that supports your vision, "I choose to eat lightly tonight," or, "I choose to cook at home instead of grabbing fast food," you are building neural pathways that support your success and make those positive choices even easier in the future.

Remember, there is nothing you **have** to do in life. There are choices and the consequences of those choices. Choose to eat food that is healthy and supportive to your body, you look and feel healthier. Choose not to and the consequences will not produce the amazing life you came here to live!

Free Yourself from Emotional Barriers Blocking Your Success

When it comes to making changes, it is vital to include one of the most important components, your emotional body. To separate our choices from our emotions is like trying to kayak rapids without getting wet. In a word, impossible!

You may be able to override your emotions in the short run, but I guarantee you, it is not sustainable. You may use your will to change certain behaviors, but if the going gets tough and the emotional body kicks in, you are driven by a force much stronger than your will.

Jane came to my office a couple of years ago complaining of overall malaise.

"I'm not sure but I think I may be having an issue with gluten."

"Why do you think that?" I inquired. "What is it you're feeling?"

"I don't know, just an overall lethargy and sort of bloated feeling."

We ran some tests and, sure enough, found she was correct; she had an intolerance to gluten.

"Okay," I said. "You were correct, so now the best course of action is to stop eating anything that contains gluten."

Grateful, she left the office, declaring herself a "gluten-free zone!"

At her next appointment, she came in fuming.

"I can't do this," she said, arms crossed and face firmly scowled. "Coming here is a waste of my time and money."

"Okay," I said cautiously, "tell me exactly what's going on."

"Well, isn't it obvious? This is crazy! You can't live in this world and not eat gluten. It's impossible!"

"Alright, let's look at the situation."

"Look all you want," she said, shifting her weight to turn away from me. "I'm not doing it."

"I hear that but, just for a minute…can you give me a minute?"

"Whatever," she mumbled, shrugging her shoulders.

"Okay, when you first came in, you told me you didn't feel well when you ate gluten products. You felt lethargic and bloated."

Silence.

I carried on. "You know it's harmful to your system and you'd feel better if you didn't eat it, so what's at the root of your not wanting to feel better?"

Because she was having such a strong reaction to something she "knew" to be true, that gluten did not make her feel well, I was certain I knew what was going on. Her frontal cortex or conscious center of her brain was no longer in control. Her emotional brain or limbic system had kicked in and was now steering the ship. I knew, from experience, it was pointless to reason with an activated limbic brain. She had already told me she didn't feel well when she ate it, she already "knew" it wasn't good for her.

That's when we went on an emotional dig and found that when I told her to stop eating gluten containing foods, the foods that made her feel bad, it triggered something in her limbic brain, reminding her nervous system of her controlling stepfather. That memory caused her nervous system to push against what I was saying rather than being able to listen to the frontal cortex, which, at its most basic level, knew she would feel better if she didn't eat the stuff. Once the subconscious trigger had been brought to the surface and cleared, it was easy for her to choose not to eat gluten anymore.

If you *know how and what* you "should" eat, are able to make temporary changes, but then fall back to old habits, you may have an emotional barrier that is sabotaging your success. Emotional barriers are common. It's a natural process that happens as we grow and learn about personal survival.

Behaviors and responses get wired into our nervous system at a very young age as we learn to adapt to stress. Unfortunately, they aren't always constructive. But because they are so ingrained, we can find ourselves under the influence of a "program" that is no longer serving us. Not listening to her stepfather may have served a purpose when she was younger, but not listening to me, the person she is paying to help her feel better, is not.

If what you have read in this book makes sense, and yet you are unable to do it, you are not a bad person with weak willpower; you most likely have just come up against an emotional barrier that is blocking your success. There are many methods for dealing with emotional barriers. In my clinic, I use a technique called Neuro Emotional Technique (NET) to help my clients reach their goals of living healthy, stress-free lives and improve their day-to-day food choices. NET is a technique that identifies and 'helps us process' information stored in our limbic brain, our emotional center, which may be influencing and sabotaging the choices we are making in our life.

However, regardless of the method used, the important point is to identify that there is an emotional barrier and do something to address it so you can achieve your goal of a healthy success-filled life.

Identify and Clear *Avoidance Behaviors*

An avoidance behavior is a defense mechanism by which people remove themselves from unpleasant situations. In other words, they use something to distract themselves from unpleasant or uncomfortable feelings. This is very common. Many of us have one form or another of an avoidance behavior. I see the effects of avoidance behaviors in my clinic almost every day. They are often what keep people from succeeding at their desired goal. Why we lose the weight only to gain it again. Why we start an exercise routine, only to stop a few weeks or months later. But nowhere do I see avoidance behaviors play a bigger role than in the choices people make around food.

A woman came in to my clinic one day for her initial visit with a bowl of cookie dough. Yes, you read that right, a bowl of cookie dough! She brought it in, she said, to show how addicted she was to it, eating it every day. She was a nursing mother and was really scared she was harming her child with the large amounts of sugar she was consuming.

So, here she was, very clear that her behavior was not constructive but unable to do anything about it even in the face of doing possible harm to her new baby.

"Would you be willing to explore this a little further?"

"Anything," she said, desperate to find her way out of her destructive behavior.

We did some emotional clearing and found there were some very deep-seated issues blocking her. She was quite beautiful and, when she was younger, had been inappropriately touched by an older male. In her mind, keeping herself heavy was essential to her survival. When she lost weight she started to get a lot more attention from men. This attention triggered an emotional reaction that was out of her conscious control, and, before she knew it, she was eating cooking dough again.

Obviously she didn't "want" to eat the bowl of cookie dough. She wanted to take the best care of her daughter that she could and knew her behavior was harmful for both of them, but her avoidance behavior was so embedded, she felt out of control of her choices. Obviously, further professional support was necessary around this issue; however, in the meantime, by making the connection between her past and her food choices in a conscious way, she was able to override the emotional trigger and make better food choices in the present.

This is not an uncommon scenario. Though the cookie dough may have been extreme, the behavior is more common than we realize. There are all kinds of avoidance behaviors from cigarette smoking to eating certain foods that are not good for us.

The ability to calm and soothe oneself under stress is a strength. The problem arises with the *how* of that self-soothing. Are we making positive choices in our self-care or are we increasing the amount of stress in the body with destructive choices?

When we make choices from a "need," we often make choices that do not really soothe us. It's like comforting oneself with a caress and then finishing off that love with a quick slap. Doing things in the name of love with a sting at the end is not actually helping you reach your goal of feeling better. Often, these behaviors are learned early in childhood as our parents tried to soothe us with ice cream or a cookie. It seemed like a good idea at the time but the long-term effects of that kind of caring are not positive when we continue to "self-soothe" in that way.

You may start to identify your own unique way of avoidance: those late-night cravings helping you not feel so lonely, that sugar you just have to have, or those glasses of wine at the end of the day to take the edge off. If you do, I encourage you to find a NET practitioner, psychologist, or other professional who can help you identify and remove the stimuli that may be keeping your avoidance behavior in place. It may be the key to you finally having success at reaching your goal of better health once and for all.

If Doing It for Yourself Is Hard, Do It for the Planet: Save Yourself, Save the Planet

You can watch all those great, painful-to-witness movies about how bad things are. You can then walk around feeling guilty that you have done nothing to help, or you can begin where all global change begins, with yourself. Start making healthful choices that serve your highest and best.

Pay attention to what you are putting in your mouth. Spend your dollars on high quality, low negative-impact foods. Make choices that will not harm you, your children, your cleaning staff, or your pets. Do this and you know what? You'll stop feeling the need to drag yourself through the guilt of all you're not doing because you will be doing a lot for yourself and, consequently, for the planet.

Remember Wal-Mart and RBST, the growth hormone used to make dairy cows produce milk 24/7? That's right: consumers stopped buying it and Wal-Mart stopped selling it. Done and done!

Every dollar spent supporting practices and businesses that supply you with good food, clean skin care, and nontoxic cleaning supplies is a dollar spent supporting our planet. It is dollar spent supporting an economy that is based on good principles instead of greed.

This is how we change the world; we change it through our moment-to-moment, day-to-day habits.

Make choices that support your health and you are having a direct effect on helping to save the health of this planet. Now, doesn't that feel good?

After the Healing Live by the 80/20 Rule

Once your body has gone through the healing phase and you are ready to live your life while maintaining your healthier level of homeostasis, I recommend the 80/20 rule.

80% of the time you live by the principles outlined in this book, and, for the other 20% of the time, go with the flow of what is happening. Remember, moderation is always best.

However, what is moderation for you may be different than for someone else. Every body is different, so determining what is moderation for you will be a trial-and-error process. If you are generally healthy, your 80/20 rule may include more than if you have health challenges. Some people may only be able to tolerate very little variations. If this is you, you will know it.

My personal 80/20 rule is a lot tighter than most people's 80/20 rule. My 20% consists of extra nuts, or raw desserts. A glass of wine and even chemical-filled food are extravagances I do not partake in.

Pay attention. Listen to your body. Develop an awareness of what your body needs. A key component to successful self-care and the most effective way to use the 80/20 rule is to stay aware.

Make conscious choices and make sure your indulgence is worth it! I would often joke with a client when they would come to see me because they were feeling awful after eating something they knew wasn't good for them by smiling and saying that was one expensive sticky bun.

When Applying the 80/20 Rule, Watch Your Overall Stress Level

When you are already under a lot of stress, it is not the time to add more stress by drinking too much alcohol or eating chemical-laden foods or adding extra sugar to your eating choices. If, however, your overall stress level is low, a little lenience will probably be fine.

Remember, common foods available in most stores increase the workload of your liver and add extra stress to the body. So when choosing to have a *Party Day*, as I like to call it, do it when things in your life are fairly calm so that your body can easily handle the added physical stress.

Oftentimes, people choose to have a party day, or two, or three when they are already under a great amount of stress. Before they know it, their level of homeostasis has dropped and they don't even notice they are starting to feel subpar again. Waking up tired and with a mild headache once again becomes normal.

For 80% of the time, take mindful care of yourself. And if you are under stress, maybe even increase that. But when things are going well, and you just want to taste that flavor you loved as a child, or have a few extra beers, by all means go ahead!

This isn't about being rigid; this is about paying attention. It's about playing it smart so you wake up when you're eighty feeling exactly how you wanted to feel instead of in some health nightmare wondering how the heck you got there.

Choose Food, Be Healthy and Thrive

> *Newton's First Law of Motion; an object at rest will remain at rest and an object in motion will remain in motion at the exact speed and direction unless acted upon by an equal and opposite force.*

Congratulations! You have made a big commitment by finishing this book. You have made a commitment to learning how you can change the way you feel, and, in making that commitment, you have taken a very important first step in that direction.

That said, ultimately, the words in this book are just ideas. They are words on a page unless acted upon.

In physics for a Law to be a law, it has to hold true in all circumstances. So, according to Newton's First Law of Motion, the trajectory of your life, the trajectory of your health will not change unless you take action. In other words, these words will have no effect on your reality, your health, your future, unless you exert a force by taking a step in a new direction.

Please, do not let this become another interesting book sitting on your shelf, collecting dust. Start with the 21-Day Diet Detox. Experience for yourself how your food choices are affecting how you feel. If the 21-Day Diet Detox feels like too much right now, then start with the work sheet in Chapter 9 in the section, Transitioning off the Diet Detox.

It does not matter how you start, as long as you take a step in a new direction. It just takes one step after another over time to get you to a completely different place. Aren't you worth that much effort? Isn't your future worth a little effort now? I know it is. I know you are worth every bit of the effort it takes to get your life and your health back in alignment with the true vision of how you dream it to be.

It is my sincerest wish that you know this too, and you prove it to yourself by taking that first step today.

END NOTES

1. "Definition of Choice, accessed August 29, 2015, http://www.brainyquote.com/words/ch/choice143602.html#bC4C mfSOEOH3mPVJ.99
2. Oxford Dictionaries, s.v. "should," accessed August 29, 2015, http://www.oxforddictionaries.com/definition/english/should

ABOUT THE AUTHOR

Cari Schaefer, M.A. TCM, L.Ac., resides in Topanga Canyon, California with her new husband and children. She has been a natural health practitioner for over 16 years, helping thousands of people improve their health and live a more vital life, using diet as a core healing tool. Cari currently runs the Sustainable Health Center in Santa Monica, California.

The expertise and wisdom shared with you in this book comes not only from Cari's nutritional education (her multidisciplinary study includes a Masters Degree in Traditional Chinese Medicine, national certification in herbalism and acupuncture, certifications in Nutrition Response Testing and Neuro Emotional Technique, and certification as a Yoga instructor) but also from her clients' and her own real-life experiences.

At age 32, Cari faced her own health crisis. When walking three blocks became challenging due to extreme fatigue, constant pain, and depression, she learned, firsthand, the devastation that poor health causes in your life and the critical role food plays in your health.

Cari shares what she has learned with others through one-on-one care, radio appearances, public speaking, workshops, and by teaching and mentoring other healthcare practitioners.

www.sustainablehc.com

INDEX

bowel movements, 42-43, 188
brain, 5, 35, 43, 206, 209
    amino acids and health of, 112
    diseases of, 66-67, 122-123
    electrolytes and functioning of, 132
    gluten and diseases of, 67, 69
    low-fat diet and, 123
    nonabsorbable minerals and plaque, 74
    pesticides and developing, 56
broken bones, 36
distilled water and, 21

C
calcium, 44, 73-74, 108-109, 129
cancer, ix, 56, 94, 100-101, 113, 115, 136, 138
celiac disease, 65-66
chemicals, 2-4, 7, 39, 54, 58-60, 77-81, 84
in artificial sweeteners, 138
    in dairy, 107-108
    in fats, 123
    in fruits and vegetables, 103
    in grains, 94-95
    in meat, 113, 115
    in processed food, 180
    in salt, 129
    in soy, 100
    in water, 133
cholesterol, 7, 19, 25-26
    eggs and, 120
    HDL and LDL, 25-26
    hydrogenated oils and, 123
coffee, 158-159, 164, 175-176, 180
corn, 61-62
    syrup, 138
cortisol, 46-49, 151-152
consumer-supported agriculture (CSA), 104, 117, 121, 156
C.R.A.P., 1-3, 7, 52, 58-60, 77
    dairy, 107-109

Made in the USA
San Bernardino, CA
01 May 2017